I0022346

Cleaning

With Essential Oil

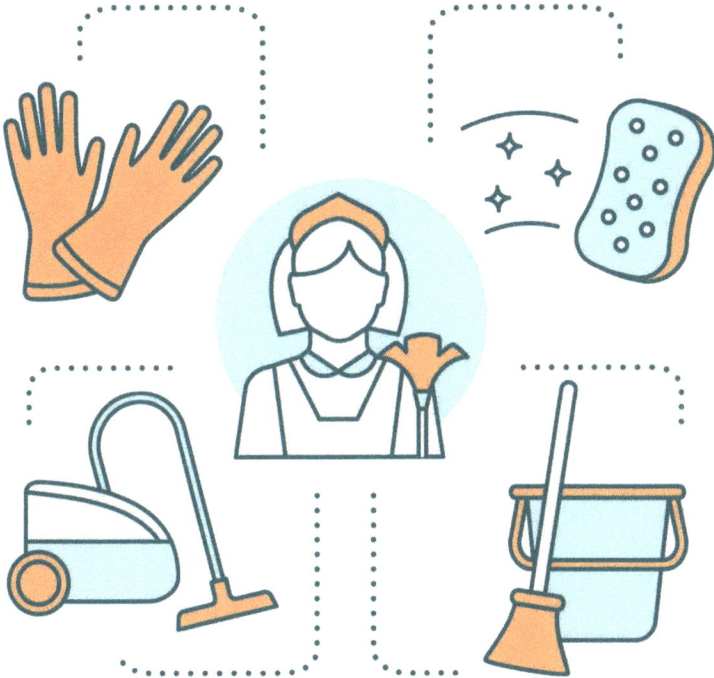

Rebecca Park Totilo

Copyright ©2019 by Rebecca Park Totilo

All rights reserved. No part of this book may be reproduced or transmitted in any form or by any means without written permission of the author.

Printed in the United States of America.

Published by Rebecca at the Well Foundation.

No part of this publication may be reproduced, stored in a retrieval system or transmitted in any form by any means—electronic, mechanical, photocopy, recording or otherwise—without written permission of the copyright holder, except as provided by USA copyright law.

Disclaimer Notice: The information contained in this book is intended for educational purposes only and is not meant to be a substitute for medical care or prescribe treatment for any specific health condition. Please see a qualified healthcare provider for medical treatment. The author and publisher assume no responsibility or liability for any person or group for any loss, damage or injury resulting from the use or misuse of any information in this book. No express or implied guarantee is given regarding the effects of using any of the products described herein.

Paperback ISBN: 978-0-9991865-5-8

Electronic ISBN: 978-0-9991865-6-5

Contents

CLEANING WITH ESSENTIAL OILS

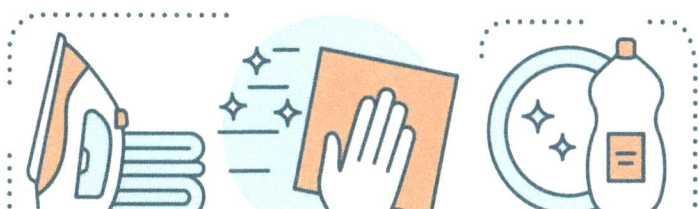

There's nothing more gratifying than entering a fresh, clean house – especially after a long and arduous day at work. Using essential oils for cleaning allows you to create a pleasant environment that not only makes your guests feel welcome and at ease when they visit but also provides a healthy home for your family to dwell in.

Of course, advertisements would have people believe that air fresheners, scented candles, and other cleaning products can accomplish this and even eliminate bad odors. Some do temporarily, but these store-bought products may also be sources of volatile organic compounds or VOCs that pose a variety of health risks due to the potentially harmful chemicals they contain.

Don't be fooled into believing that only these harsh chem-

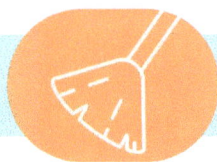

icals can get the job done and sanitize your household surfaces. Essential oils not only can get rid of unpleasant odors (even if you own pets or live with a smoker), they can handle just about all of the dirty jobs around the house. This includes using essential oils to clean everything from surfaces, floors, and windows, wash and dry your laundry, clean and deodorize your carpets, drapes, or window coverings, neutralize cooking odors, and disinfect kitchen appliances and countertops.

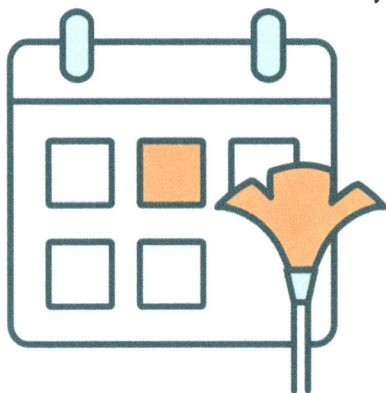

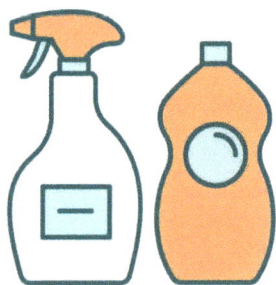

If you are already an avid user of essential oils, cleaning and maintaining your home using natural ingredients such as essential oils is a no-brainer! You can easily replace expensive cleaners with homemade products using the essential oils you have on hand for only pennies. What a more economical and environmentally friendly way to go! Plus, they smell SO much better!

WHY CLEAN WITH ESSENTIAL OILS?

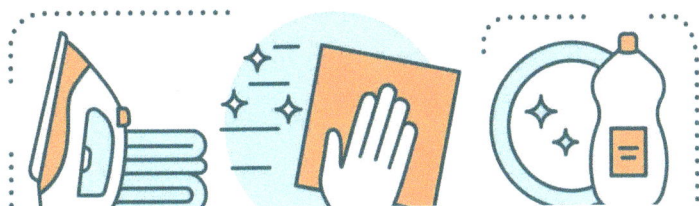

Have you ever wondered what Martha Stewart's house might smell like?

People magazine reported in a November 2016 article that Martha Stewart does not like "Stinky Homes."

E ven if you haven't, imagine for a moment the smell of fresh-baked cookies, expansive, cedar-lined closets, and fresh flowers in every room. It's easy to visualize the fresh-cut flowers or see the lavender swaying in the breeze outside along the wrap porch at her estate on Martha's Vineyard.

You could create a gorgeous garden of hydrangeas and beautiful flowers and have fresh-cut arrangements on your

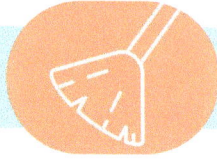

kitchen table daily too, but if you're like me, you don't have the budget or time for that. So instead, a great way to get that fresh "signature aroma" in your home is to start cleaning with essential oils. As you use essential oils for cleaning, you will be able to enjoy the amazing aroma they emit and fill your home with an uplifting and invigorating scent that can last for hours.

> *Cleaning Tip: Cleaning with essential oil makes your house smell amazing!*

By the way, if you ever plan on inviting Martha over for brunch, follow her advice: "Nix the overpowering laundry detergents, don't spray too much room spray in one place, and above all, don't mix too much of a good thing. Stick to one scent at a time," she advises. "We wouldn't want it to be the holidays and have this beautiful Winter Evergreen in one room and then Fig in another; you're going to confuse people and yourself."

A sparkling clean and spotless home is the dream of every homeowner. Having an immaculate home need not be overly expensive, requiring a professional cleaning service. With green cleaners, you can have a clean, serene, and

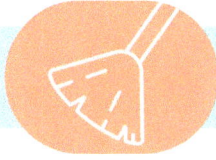

inspiring home to come back to after a long day. Besides making your own cleaners because it's simple and afford-able, green cleaners have a plethora of advantages over other types of synthetic cleaners. Their bio-degradable properties make them eco-friendly and less harmful both to the user and the product com-pared to a synthetic detergent, which is more toxic than the germs it is supposed to de-stroy. Like many other natural products, green cleaners can be relied on to be effective, and science has proven that green cleaners are more effective and leave soothing, sat-isfying, and refreshing aura.

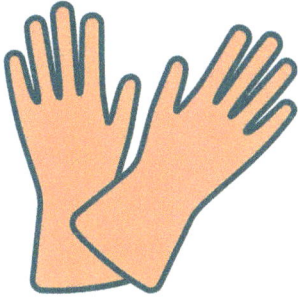

Cleaning With Essential Oils Is Better For Your Health

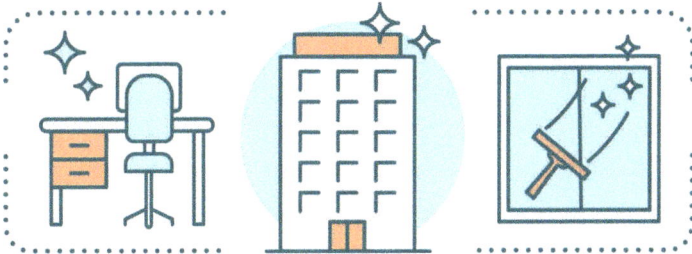

When it comes to improving our health, we tend to focus

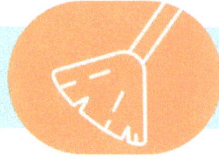

on nutrition and exercise, while focusing less on our environment, which could be affecting our overall wellbeing. Creating a clean environment to retreat to is an integral part of a healthy lifestyle, while an unclean, unkempt home could have a negative impact on your health and ultimately lead to serious health consequences.

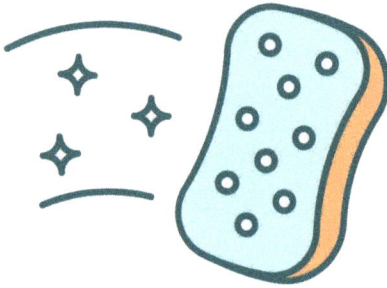

If you're still using conventional products with harmful, hormone-disrupting chemicals, it's time to ditch those and switch to all-natural cleaning products with essential oils; add essential oils to clean your laundry, sanitize your kitchen, and nix the mold in your bathroom shower – all with the confidence of knowing these active cleaning agents won't harm your health.

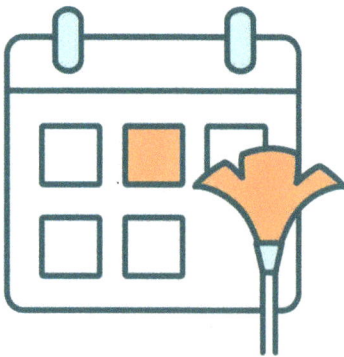

If you are already using essential oils, you may know they are packed with potent antioxidants and have versatile health benefits. As you're cleaning

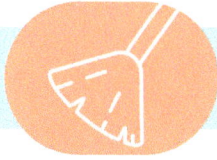

your home, you'll be inhaling the aroma of these powerful drops. You can increase your energy, improve circulation, support respiratory health, bust bacteria, boost your immune system, improve your mood, support your hormones and more – the list goes on!

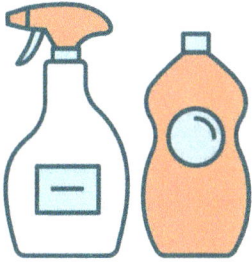

For people who suffer from allergies or are sensitive to synthetic fragrances, it is especially important to avoid harsh chemicals and look for healthy alternatives. Recent studies have shown that synthetic fragrances can be irritating to the skin and, in some cases, have immune-toxic and neurotoxic effects on the body. Over time, this can wreak havoc on the immune system and cause health issues down the road.

Using essential oils in cleaning products offers a natural solution that safeguards your family's health while minimizing the impact on the environment. As a safer alternative to harsh chemicals for scrubbing and cleaning, essential oils can be used in conjunction with other natural products such as baking soda and vinegar that are bio-

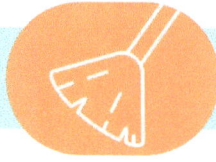

degradable and will not add toxins to the water and soil. These small changes in the way you clean your home can make a difference on our planet.

Cleaning With Essential Oils Is Better For Your Wallet

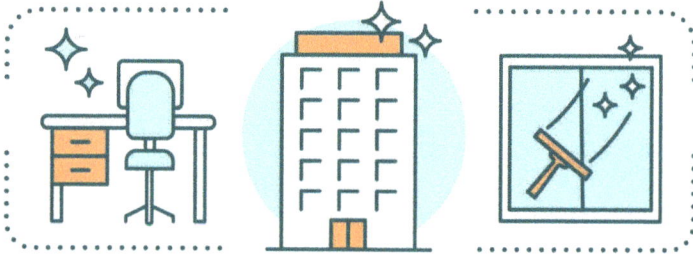

Of course, essential oils are great for cleaning because they can save you money! Have you ever looked at the prices for natural cleaners in health food stores? Let's face it: commercial natural cleaning products are expensive. When you make a small batch of cleaners at home using essential oils, you'll be spending only a fraction of what their store-bought commercial counterparts cost. Plus, only a tiny amount will be needed, usually only a few drops for most cleaning appli-

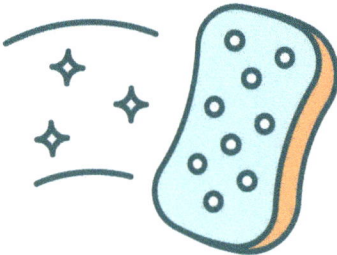

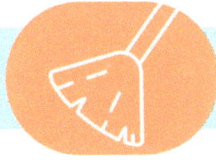

cations due to their potency. That small bottle of oil will go a long way toward keeping your house clean! So whether you're interested in a more natural way or a less expensive way to clean your home, cleaning with essential oils can help!

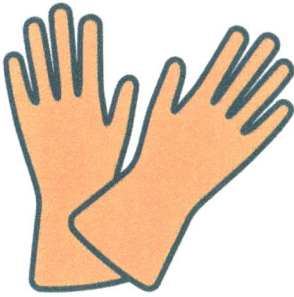

Not only can you make household cleaners (and really you only need a few to cover most cleaning jobs), but you can also use your essential oil for other uses. Can you say versatility? The same lemon essential oil that can be used to scrub out the sink is also perfect to add to your water bottle throughout the day to increase hydration and gently stimulate the lymphatic system to flush toxins.

Cleaning With Essential Oil Works

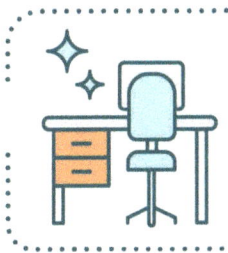

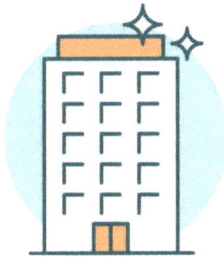

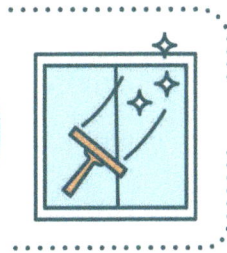

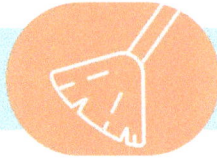

One of the most obvious reasons for using essential oils in your cleaning products is that they really work! Many essential oils not only have grease-cutting and stain-fighting abilities, but they also have antimicrobial properties that kill viruses, bacteria, and fungi. Because of these special properties, essential oils can be used as a safe and natural alternative to the chemicals found in commercial cleaning products. With natural cleansing properties, essential oils provide a simple yet powerful way to keep things sparkling.

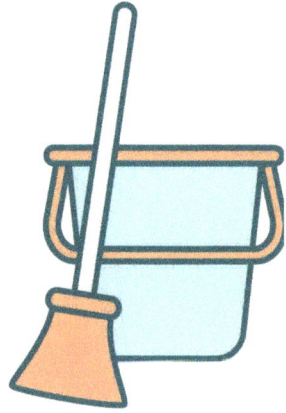

Cleaning Tip: *Buyer Beware*

Most commercial cleaning products are loaded with artificial coloring, fragrances, and harsh cleaning agents like bleach, ammonia, and more. This is why people prefer using natural products because they want to know exactly what is in their products due to safety con-

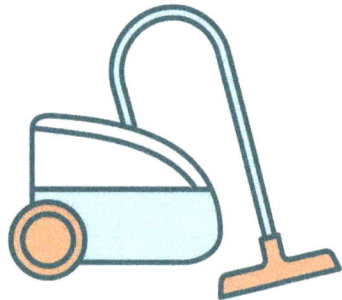

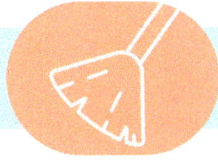

cerns. It is a known fact that store-bought chemical-laden products can cause air pollution by off-gassing toxic fumes. These fumes can irritate your eyes, nose, and respiratory system. Young family members and pets are most at risk.

WHAT ARE ESSENTIAL OILS?

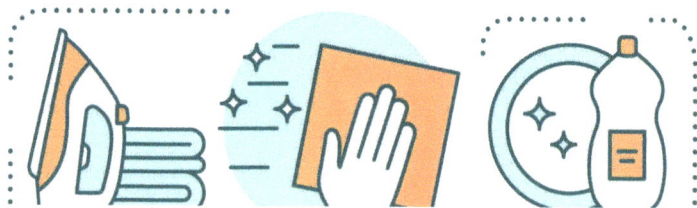

Essential oils are highly concentrated liquids that contain volatile aroma compounds found in special glands of specific plants. These cells and glands that house the essential oil are found in different parts of different plants. For instance, essential oils may come from the petals of a rose, the rind of a lemon, or the seeds or leaves of the herb cilantro.

Cleaning Tip: Essential oils should not be confused with perfume or fragrance oils.

You have probably walked past "aromatherapy candles" with their strong aroma wafting through the aisle with the words "contains essential oils." But the big question is: Do these candles contain real essential oils or fragrance oils?

Real essential oils are "oils" that have been extracted from

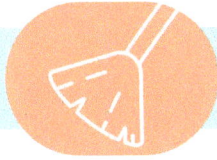

various species of flowers, fruits, herbs, leaves, seeds, resin, stems, roots, and bark of botanicals. The oils from these natural sources are pure, which means they are not made from synthetic materials in a laboratory like fragrance oils. On the other hand, fragrance oils are primarily made with synthetic chemicals to achieve the scents used in candles and bath and body products. Scents such as "pumpkin spice" are not necessarily derived from "pumpkins" and "spices," but synthetic blends of chemicals that are combined to achieve the desired scent. Fragrance oil manufacturers are not required to disclose the various ingredients used but are required to list harmful chemicals on the Material and Safety Data Sheet.

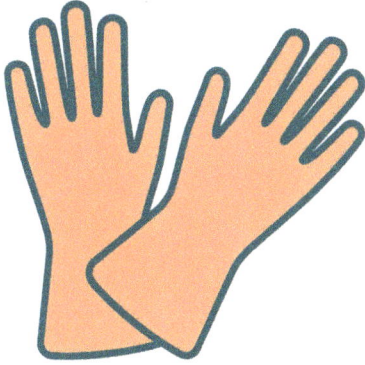

Essential oils are extracted from botanical material by one of four methods:

- Steam distillation: Heat is used to draw out essential oils. This is the most common method used today.

- Cold press extraction: This method removes oils from

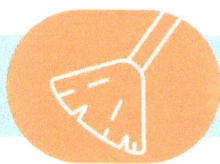

the skins of fruits without damage from heat.

- Chemical solvent extraction: This method uses solvents such as alcohol to extract harder-to-get essential oils.

- Effleurage method: This method involves using odorless fats or oils to absorb the perfume of fresh-cut flowers.

Depending on which extraction process used, one pound of essential oil can require hundreds of pounds of plant matter. For instance, it takes roughly 200 pounds of lavender flowers to produce one pound of lavender oil. The remaining plant material of lavender flowers may be used for other purposes such as soap additives, teas, and pillows. Just think about this when you are buying a bottle of lavender essential oil; you are actually purchasing the essence of quite a few lavender flowers!

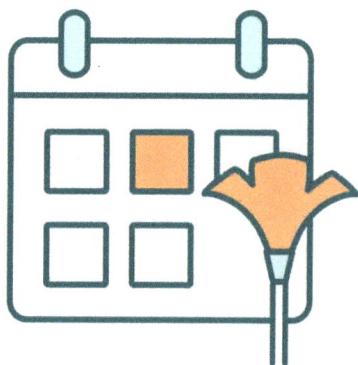

Through distillation, these aromatic substances are extracted and bottled. The steam water that runs off during the distillation process, which contains approximately 2%

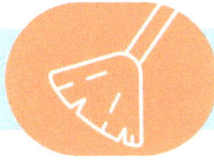

dilution of essential oil, is called "hydrosol." Hydrosols are also beneficial and can be used to clean your floors or as a substitute for water in some of your cleaning products.

Contrary to essential oils being called "oils," they do not have an oily feel at all. The majority of them are clear, but there are some that are amber or yellow in color. The color varies depending on the type of plant the oil came from.

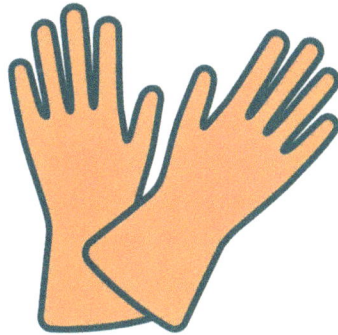

Different parts of the plant used for distillation include petals, seeds, stems, bark, leaves, or roots. While different methods of extraction are used, the most common is steam distillation. Some other methods include carbon dioxide extraction, pressing, and solvent extraction.

Each essential oil contains a unique set of chemical components, and thus, its own set of benefits. Depending on which plant the oil comes from, the combination of chemical con-

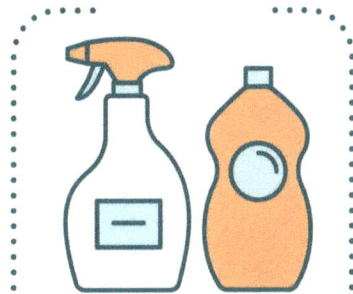

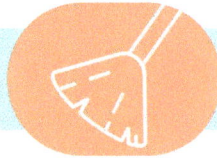

stituents in any essential oil can vary. Essential oils containing the highest percentage of chemical properties that can provide cleansing benefits and act as natural cleansing agents will be the most effective for household cleaning.

In the summary below, you can see the chemical constituents that contain cleansing properties and which essential oils contain the highest concentration of these.

Aldehydes

Known for their citrus-like and powerful fragrance, aldehydes such as cinnamaldehyde and geranial are frequently found in essential oils. Aldehydes can also be strongly antifungal, antiviral, and antiseptic, although they may cause skin irritation.

Oils high in aldehydes beneficial for cleaning include cassia, cilantro, cinnamon, citronella, eucalyptus, lemongrass, and melissa.

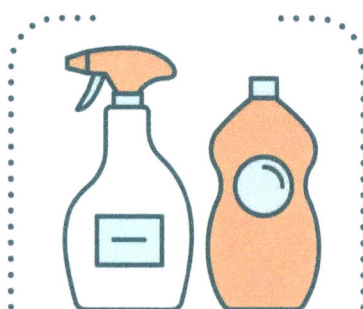

Monoterpenes

Found in most essential oils, monoterpenes are hydrocarbons with numerous benefits. Around 90% of citrus oils

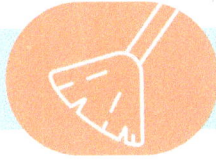

contain limonene, which can kill viruses. Although they can be potential skin irritants, monoterpenes have many positive cleansing abilities – they are generally antibacterial and antiseptic.

Oils high in monoterpenes beneficial for cleaning include bergamot, cypress, grapefruit, juniper berry, lemon, lime, pine, silver fir, tea tree, and orange.

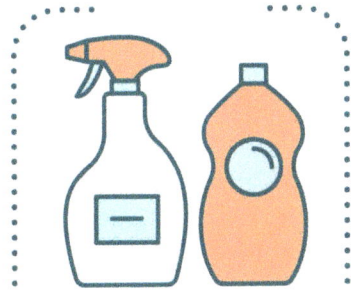

Phenols

Phenols are known to be powerful surface cleansers and effec¬tive at both killing and preventing the growth of bacteria, fungi, and viruses. Phenols commonly found in essential oils include antheole, carvacrol, eugenol, and thymol. Due to their strength, phenols can be extremely irritating to the skin and are known as "hot oils" due to the burning sensation they can produce on the skin.

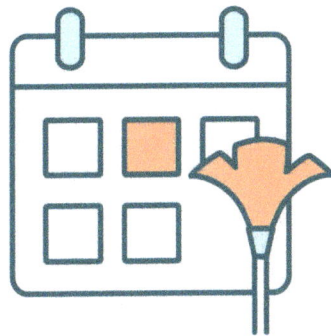

Oils high in phenols beneficial for cleaning include basil,

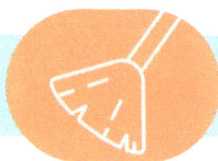

clove, thyme, peppermint, oregano, and wintergreen.

All essential oils are antibacterial to some extent, but some also have antiviral and antifungal properties that are beneficial as surface cleaning agents. Not only will they out-perform their chemical and synthetic counterparts, but in the long run they will also be safer and more pleasant for you and everyone in your home.

Essential Oil Cleaning Properties

Knowing which essential oils to use when cleaning can be tricky if you don't know what they can do. Here is a short list of some the properties to look for when deciding which to clean with.

Antibacterial: Bay, camphor, cardamom, chamomile, citronella, cypress, eucalyptus, ginger, juniper, lavender, lemon, lemongrass, lemon verbena, lime, marjoram, orange, pine, rosemary, sage, sandalwood, spearmint, tea tree, thyme, wintergreen

Antiviral: Cinnamon, clove, eucalyptus, lavender, lemon, oregano, sandalwood, tea tree, thyme

Antifungal: Eucalyptus, juniper, lavender, lemon, patchouli, sage, sandalwood, savory, tea tree, thyme

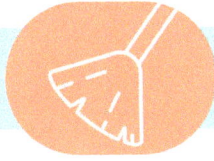

Antibiotic: Bergamot, chamomile, clove, eucalyptus, lavender, lemon, lime, nutmeg, oregano, patchouli, pine, tea tree

Cleaning Tip: *Cleansing Properties*

Essential oils that have cleansing properties include lemon, eucalyptus, pine, clove, juniper berry, rosemary, thyme, oregano and tea tree, to name a few. Many of these oils have the added benefit of acting as insect repellents as well, keeping your home free of unwanted pests while others can be used as disinfectants due to their potent antimicrobial ability in destroying microorganisms.

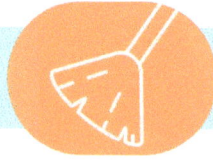

WHICH ESSENTIAL OILS ARE GOOD FOR CLEANING?

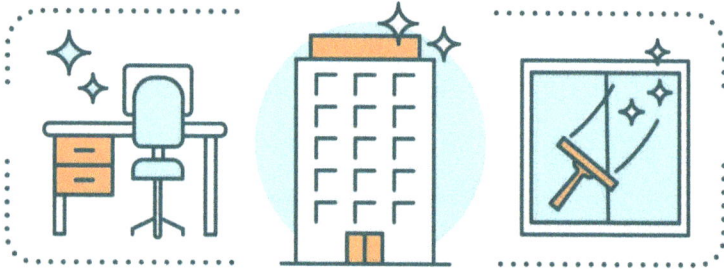

Choosing which essential oils to use for cleaning will depend on your personal preference for a particular scent, the quality of the essential oil you're using, which cleaning properties the essential oil contains, and how it will be used.

Cleaning Tip: Four Must-Have Essential Oils for Cleaning

Some oils have antibacterial qualities while others have antifungal qualities; some have both. It's good to know the cleaning properties and benefits of the various oils you

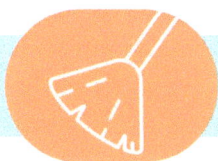

may use. That way you're not using an essential oil that contains antibacterial properties when you want to be using an essential oil that has antifungal properties.

These four oils are a must-have for your natural cleaning arsenal!

- *Tea Tree Essential Oil* has antibacterial, antiviral, and antifungal properties, which makes it very useful for killing germs on just about any surface in your home. It's very useful during cold and flu season for eliminating germs on frequently touched objects like doorknobs, countertops, and other common hard and soft surfaces.

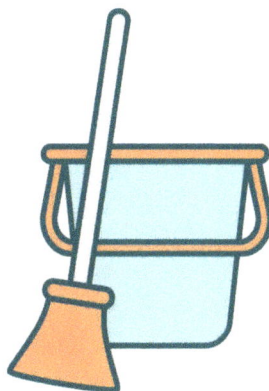

- *Lavender Essential Oil* has antimicrobial properties with a floral fragrance that has been shown to have a relaxing effect. Use it to keep fabrics and textiles around your house clean and fresh!

- *Lemon Essential Oil* is antibacterial and can cut through greasy messes with ease! It's an excellent choice for

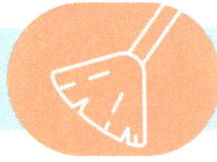

cleaning jobs in the kitchen, like your stovetop, oven, and even your floors.

- *Peppermint Essential Oil* has antibacterial qualities, with a minty fresh scent that has an invigorating effect. This oil makes a great all-purpose cleaner for just about any surface in your house!

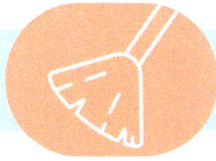

TOP TEN ESSENTIAL OILS FOR CLEANING

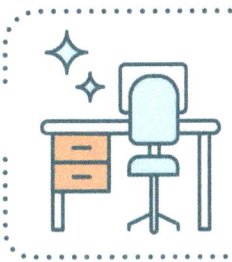

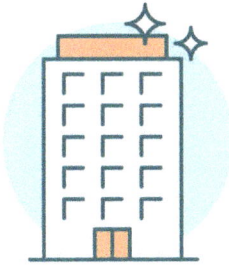

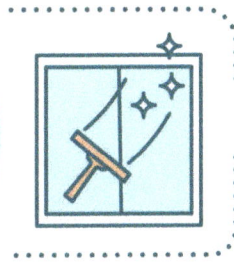

1. LEMON

This citrusy, light essential oil brings a powerful punch to homemade cleaning recipes with its antibacterial and antiviral components. Because of its surface cleansing properties, lemon essential oil works to sanitize, degrease and remove stubborn stains. In the kitchen, lemon oil can be used to deodorize your fridge or mop the floor. To use as a polish, combine ten drops with ½ cup olive oil. Rub in with a soft cloth to remove smudges and fingerprints and bring out the beauty in wood furniture.

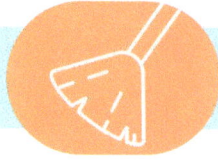

2. TEA TREE (MELALEUCA)

For thousands of years, tea tree has been used because of its powerful antimicrobial action against infectious organisms, including bacteria, viruses, and fungi. This miracle oil is known to do just about anything. When added to recipes for cleaning products such as homemade disinfectant wipes, it offers protection from germs while tackling quick cleanups. In the bathroom, tea tree essential oil can be used in shower cleaners to prevent mold and mildew from growing along tile crevices and in DIY daily shower sprays without leaving the harsh chemical residue. As a handy weapon against insects, tea tree oil can be used in a spray bottle with water to keep flies, fleas, and other annoying pests away.

3. ROSEMARY

In ancient times, rosemary leaves were burned to purify the air in hospitals. Today, the essential oil extends its antimicrobial and antibacterial activities as a superb addition to any cleaner for the kitchen or bath. Its strong herbaceous aroma blends well with other oils for homemade disinfectant sprays or as a diffuser blend during flu season. Rose-

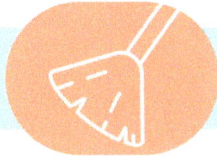

mary and lemon essential oils are a winning combination to diffuse when you may be coping with stress and need to see things from a clearer perspective.

4. ORANGE

With so many uses in the home, orange essential oil could easily be considered the multi-tool of oils. Like other citrus oils, it contains limonene, a natural cleansing compound that is often used in many commercial cleaning products. Orange essential oil in a diffuser or room spray brightens a room up with its perky, sweet fragrance. It is also effective as a degreaser, removing sticky substances from surfaces, plus it can be used on stainless steel appliances, floors, and more.

5. LAVENDER

Lavender, nature's antibacterial, is considered one of the most popular fragrances to create a mood. As a gentle oil, it is safe for most surfaces. For cleaning, add 4 to 5 drops of lavender to vinegar and use as needed. For laundry, use in a linen spray, or add to a dishwashing liquid for washing dishes.

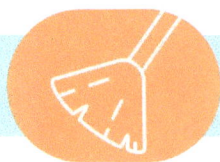

6. EUCALYPTUS

As a natural deodorizer, eucalyptus is a great deterrent for pests in kitchen cupboards. It also comes in handy for scouring the stovetop as a powerful grease buster. When added to baking soda, eucalyptus can be used to dry clean carpets, mattresses, and stuffed toys. For the bathroom, use as a toilet disinfectant by adding several drops in the bowl. Place several drops on a hot, damp cloth and wipe down surfaces to prevent mold and mildew.

7. PEPPERMINT

With its crisp, invigorating scent and powerful antibacterial properties, peppermint makes a great addition to homemade spray cleaners and natural deodorizing sprays. For creepy crawly pests such as silverfish and centipedes, place several drops of peppermint essential oil in places that collect moisture: basements, under cabinets, or in garages. To stop ants in their tracks, wipe your cabinets with a damp sponge and 6 to 8 drops of peppermint essential oil. Place several drops on windowsills, along woodwork, and in corners.

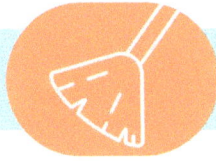

8. CINNAMON

Cinnamon has been recognized for its amazing benefits in the kitchen and is beneficial for its antifungal and antimicrobial properties. This oil is a powerful agent against mold and makes an excellent addition to a DIY mold and mildew spray. Most people love the smell of cinnamon, which works well as an air freshener in a room spray. Cinnamon oil is another oil good as a pest deterrent and can be added to a lotion as a natural and safe insect repellent. To use indoors for pest control, add several drops of oil to a cotton ball and place in window sills or where needed.

9. PINE

As a popular ingredient in floor cleaners, pine essential oil is used as a disinfectant, sanitizer, and microbicide because of its ability to kill yeast spores, E.coli bacteria and other household germs. Pine oil works to purify the air in disinfectants and room sprays, as well as rids the bathroom of mold and mildew. Pine oil can be used in a homemade floor cleaner for polishing hardwood floors, leaving a natural, fresh shine.

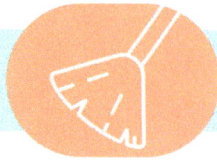

10. THYME

Thyme, one of nature's most potent essential oils against pathogens such as salmonella and E. coli, works well in the kitchen for keeping countertops clean and sanitizing cutting boards used for raw meat. Because of thyme's higher percentage of the active ingredient thymol, germs can't survive in its presence. This oil can be added to any homemade product that calls for strong antibacterial properties such as dishwashing liquid or hand soap.

Finding the right combination of essential oils to use in your cleaning products will maximize their effectiveness in disinfecting and brightening surfaces, killing mold and mildew, and preventing bacteria from creeping in, as well as offer you healthy benefits while using them.

Cleaning Tip: *Using an Essential Oil Blend*

Essential oils are sold either as pure oil, which is oil derived from only one kind of plant, or as a blend, which includes several different oils from different plant species. Buying essential oil blends saves you from having to purchase each

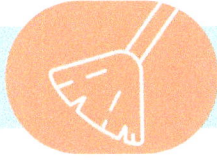

one separately, and then mix them yourself. However, when wanting more control over the fragrance and cleaning value for making household products from the recipes in this book, you will want to have all of the oils individually.

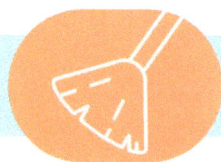

SAFETY PRECAUTIONS FOR ESSENTIAL OILS

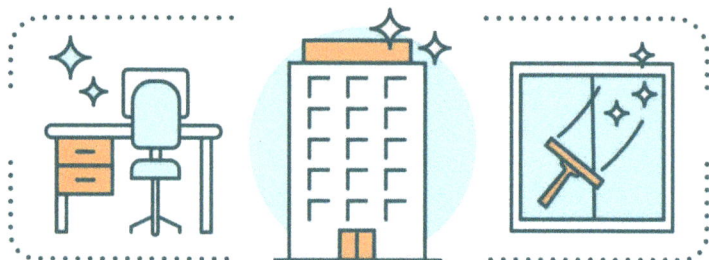

Are you new to oils? Are you wondering how to use them? Follow these safety guidelines when working with essential oils for the first time (all oil lovers can review these important reminders too).

Essential oils are powerful and should be treated like medicine – with extreme caution and care. Just like medications that have long inserts to tell you what "could happen" when you take them, we need to be educated and smart about how we handle essential oils. But, we don't have to worry and be afraid to use them. We just need to make sure we know the right way to use them and understand the precautions.

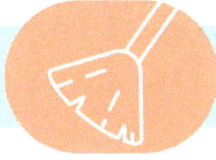

- Essential oils are powerful and, when distilled correctly, incredibly beneficial. But keep concentration levels in mind. Only use a small amount when cleaning around the house. You can always add more if needed.

- One drop of peppermint is exuivalent to 28 cups of peppermint tea. It is wonderful to get that super-charged benefit in such a small drop, but you need to be cautious as well. Not all oils are created equal! There are different levels of quality and purity. It is critical that you know what you are using.

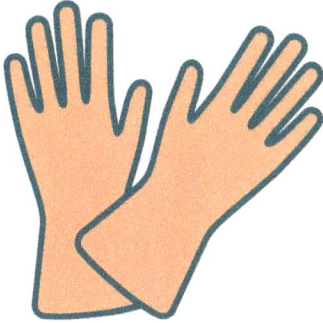

- Because of an essential oil's concentrated nature, always dilute oils before placing on skin, especially when using with children. A carrier oil such as jojoba, grapeseed, or fractionated coconut oil is recommended.

- Do not put oils in the eyes, ears, or nose. If you get oils in your eyes or on a sensitive area, flush with a

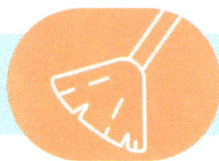

carrier oil (coconut oil, olive oil, etc.) and NOT water!

- If you experience redness or itchiness, place olive oil (or any carrier oil) on the affected area and cover with a soft cloth. The olive oil acts as an absorbent fat and binds to the essential oil, diluting its strength and allowing it to be immediately removed.

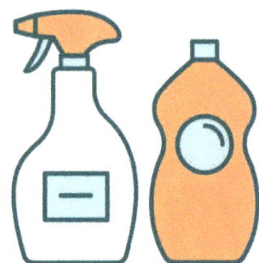

- Do not place oils in plastic cups, bottles, or containers. It will degrade the plastic. (FYI: oils can also pull the varnish off your wood furniture, so do not put your bottles down on your nice wood table!)

- Avoid use of peppermint, eucalyptus, rosemary, and wintergreen around children under age 2, particularly when sleeping, as it affects breathing.

- Some oils are not safe for use during pregnancy or if you have a history of seizures. Do your research and consult a qualified aromatherapist or healthcare

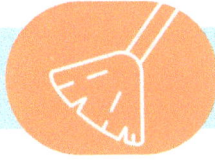

provider before use.

- Avoid prolonged use of the same oil in the same location.

- Some oils should never be used in candles, body products or diffusers. Certain oils can cause severe irritation or provoke an allergic reaction. Please consult with your physician if irritation occurs.

- Store essential oils and cleaning products out of the reach of children.

MAKING YOUR CLEANING SOLUTIONS AT HOME

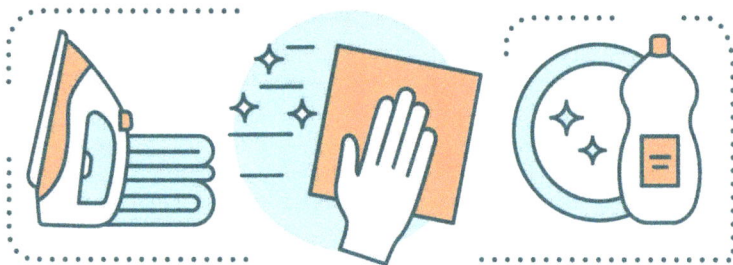

When it comes to making your natural cleaning solutions, there are several methods for incorporating essential oils into them. The amount of essential oil you add to your products will depend on the particular job at hand, what type of surface you are cleaning, and the severity of the mess you are cleaning. For routine chores around the house, you will only need to use a small amount of essential oil and other natural ingredients. Doing simple tasks around the home will call for less oil as opposed to tougher jobs where grease and grime are involved.

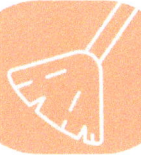

HOW MANY DROPS OF OIL SHOULD I USE?

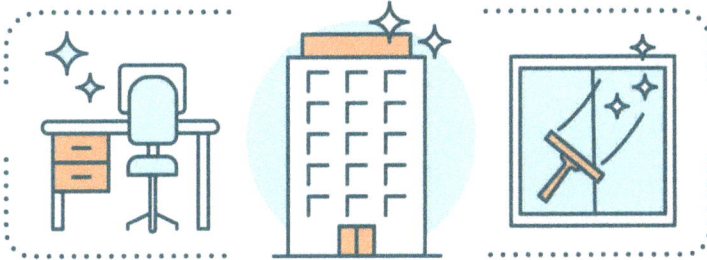

Follow this simple guide for how much essential oil to add to your DIY cleaners.

- **For simple cleaning jobs** like wiping countertops, use three drops of essential oil per cup of cleaning solution (i.e., water, vinegar, etc.).

- **For tougher jobs** like stains or grease and grime that require scrubbing, use five drops of essential oil per cup of cleaning product (i.e., baking soda, vinegar, etc.).

- **For your toughest jobs** like carpet cleaning, use 25 drops of essential oil. Keep in mind this amount will

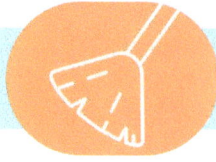

allow the scent to penetrate and be potent. Be sure to check fabrics and carpets for colorfastness before use.

Check Before Use

Be sure to test your essential oil or cleaning solution in a small, hidden area before applying a significant amount directly on a surface. This way, you will be able to see how it will react to certain fabrics, woods, and other surfaces.

Cleaning Tip: *Oil and Water Don't Mix*

After storing your essential oil cleaning products away for a while, you will notice that the oil and water will separate in your cleaning solutions. Shake vigorously before use to ensure effective cleaning.

Try to use the essential oils you have on hand. If you need others, invest in a few at a time, along with the tools and supplies you will need. Wash and reuse empty containers from old products, if possible.

Be sure to label all products with the product name (be creative!) and the list of ingredients. To ensure the ink doesn't run, purchase waterproof labels or cover the label with

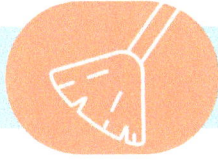

clear shipping tape to prevent smearing.

Here is a list of the ingredients you will want to have on hand for making your natural cleaning products.

NATURAL INGREDIENTS FOR MAKING CLEANING PRODUCT

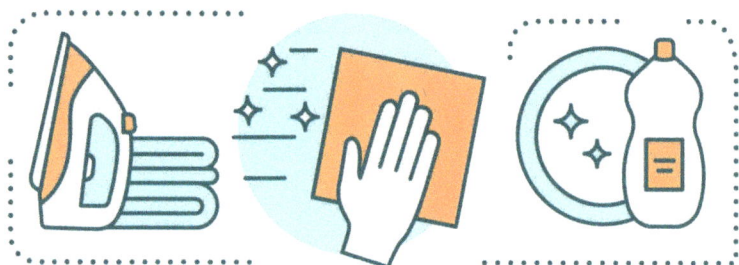

Making your own green cleaners has never been easier! All you need are a few basic ingredients that can be found at your local grocery store – and some you may already have on hand.

Baking Soda (*Sodium Bicarbonate*) – A natural, non-toxic abrasive that can be used to polish and scrub. Baking soda has a high pH and is a natural and effective deodorizer. It can be used straight out of the box as a scouring powder or all-purpose cleaner.

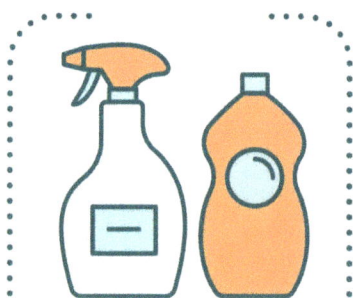

Borax (*Sodium Borate*) – Borax is the common name for the natural mineral compound sodium borate. It eliminates

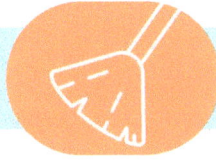

odors, removes dirt, and is antifungal and a disinfectant. Use with care around children and pets, as it may be toxic if swallowed. You can find 20 Mule Team Borax in the aisle with the laundry detergents, near the washing soda.

Citric Acid – This is a weak organic acid that removes hard water stains and is used to soften water. You'll find it health food stores, but you can even use unsweetened lemonade, which is high in citric acid.

Castile Soap, Liquid – A very mild, but highly effective all-purpose cleaner, grease-cutter, and disinfectant. Liquid castile soap is made from plant oils like coconut, jojoba or olive, rather than animal fat or synthetic substances. The pure nature of this soap means a lesser environmental impact due to reduced waste stream during manufacture and also faster biodegradability.

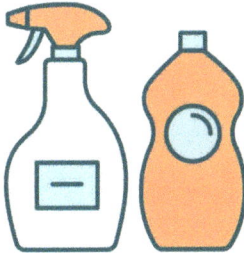

Club Soda – Stain remover and polisher.

Cornstarch – The starch of the corn obtained from corn kernels. It is non-abrasive and great for absorbing grease,

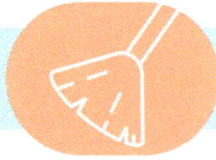

cleaning glass and freshening carpets.

Distilled Water – Distilled water is the best carrier and dirt solvent. Tap water often contains salts and minerals that can lead to spotting and build-up.

Hydrogen Peroxide (3%) – Use this product in place of ammonia and chlorine bleach. It is a stain remover and powerful disinfectant.

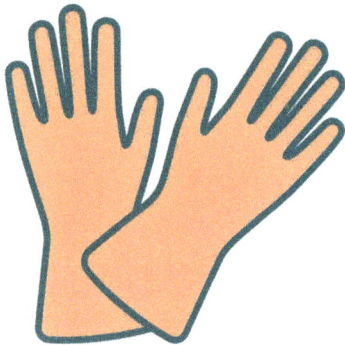

Hydrosols – Hydrosols (also known as hydrolase, distillate water, or floral waters) are the aromatic water that results from steam distilling plant materials. They are not as aromatically strong as essential oils and are very gentle. They can be used undiluted to clean any surface, added to misting bottles to be used as an air freshener, and used on all surfaces. They are perfect for cleaning floors where children and animals spend a lot of time.

Jojoba Wax (*Simmondsia Chinensis*) – Jojoba is a natural liquid wax that protects wood finishes against daily wear. It

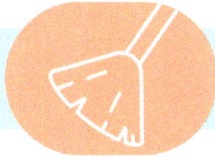

cleans, shines, and conditions wood and helps prevent drying and cracking. Use on furniture, cabinets, and paneling. Avoid on wood floors – it will make them slippery!

Salt (*Sodium Chloride*) – Regular table salt, not road salt. This item is not only inexpensive and great for removing rust, but it's also an excellent abrasive for cleaning metals like cast iron. Lemon juice and salt will shine metals like copper or steel. You can clean wine and coffee stains with hot water, salt, and vinegar.

Vinegar, White (*Acetic Acid*) – An antifungal acid that kills germs and bacteria and will stop mold and mildew in its tracks. It naturally whitens and is an excellent grease-cutter, removes soap residue, and disinfects. Vinegar is non-toxic and doesn't leave a residue. The aroma fades quickly. Use to clean hardwood, vinyl, or linoleum floors. Use the plain white vinegar and not the apple cider variety. Since it is an acid, do not use it on stone or marble, as it may etch the surface.

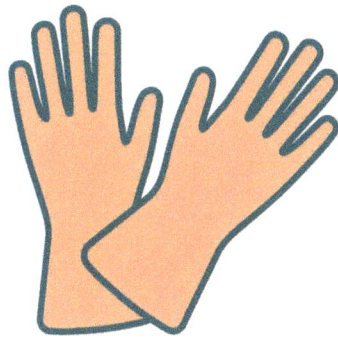

Washing Soda (*Sodium Carbonate*) – This highly alkaline

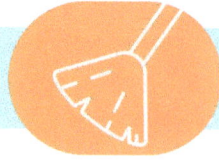

compound, also known as soda ash, is used to remove stubborn stains from laundry, cut grease, and disinfect. Don't confuse washing soda with baking soda or washing powder, which is a powdered soap used as a detergent. Arm & Hammer Super Washing Soda can be found in the laundry aisle of your supermarket.

Any of the cleaning agents above can be combined with essential oils for various cleaning tasks throughout the home.

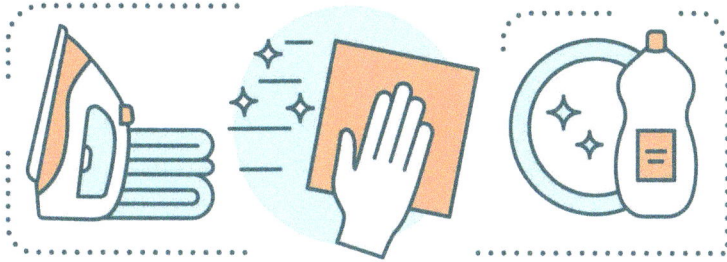

Cleaning Supplies

- Broom
- Caddy for storing cleaners and rags
- Cotton Rags
- Dustpan
- Foaming Soap Container with pump
- Funnel
- Mason Jars / Wide mouth jars with lids
- Measuring Cup
- Mixing Bowl
- Plastic Spray Bottles (or several repurposed glass cleaner bottles with sprayers)
- Rubber Gloves

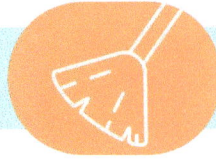

- Scrub Brush (with natural bristle)

- Spatula

- Sponge Mop

- Spray Bottle (glass)

- Squirt Floor Cleaner (repurposed swifter bottle)

- Old Toothbrushes

- Toilet Brush

Essential Oil Supplies

Having the necessary equipment available such as bottles, droppers, and containers will be a must before making your cleaning products. Below is a list of the tools you will need to get started:

- *Coffee Cans* with Lids are great for storing waxes and pastes.

- *Cloths (soft cotton)* or even rags or old t-shirts will work for dusting, polishing, making dryer sheets, and more. Using these instead of paper towels will save you money and help save the environment, too. Natural cellulose cloths are great to use since they are super absorbent and won't scratch surfaces.

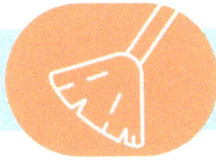

- *Large Labels* for all products with names, ingredients, how to use, and the date the products were made. If you know the expiration date, write that down.

- *Misters* with a pump, squirt, or spray top work well for linen sprays, room sprays, and plant waterers. You can find these at the dollar store.

- *Plastic Bottles* with a pump, squirt, or screw-off top are suitable for liquid soaps, shower sprays, and soft scrubs. You can find these in 2-ounce, 4-ounce, and 8-ounce sizes.

- *Plastic or Glass Spray Bottles* are great to have on hand when mak¬ing room sprays, linen spritzers or cleaning solutions. You will find these in 1-ounce, 2-ounce, 4-ounce, 8-ounce, and 16-ounce sizes.

- *Plastic Transfer Pipettes* come in different sizes and lengths for easy and precise drop measuring. They are ideal for filling small vials and for measuring small amounts of oils. Use these when you want to transfer oil from a large bottle into smaller bottles. They are for one-time use and should be thrown

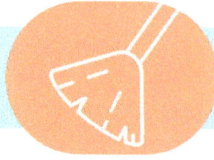

away to avoid cross-contamination.

- *Plastic Spice Shakers* with a shaker top are great for carpet fresheners and dry mattress cleaners. You can find these at the dollar store.

- *Ziploc Bags (gallon size)* will come in handy for cleaning showerheads. You can find these at the grocery store.

- *Wide-Mouth Jars with lids* come in plastic and glass. These are great for storing dishwasher pods, dryer sheets, and more. These can be purchased at the grocery store or another general supply store.

You will need waterproof labels for your bottles, and you will want them in all shapes and sizes. Visit Online Labels for a wide variety of sizes at http://www.onlinelabels.com/.

Items such as bottles and pipettes are available online at SKS Bottle & Packaging and Rachel's Supply.

WAYS TO USE ESSENTIAL OILS FOR CLEANING

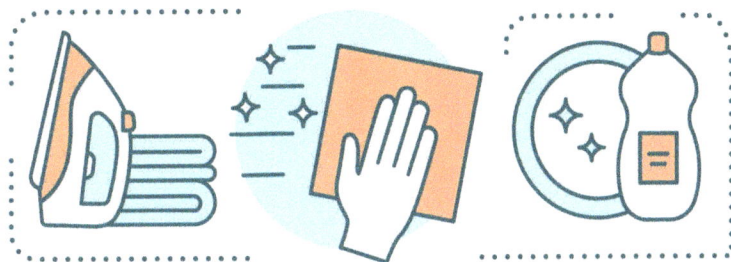

Diffusing Essential Oils

Diffusing essential oils is one of the healthiest and most efficient ways to fragrance a room or space. Depending on the type of diffuser you use, it can be the most effective, non-toxic way to eliminate odors and airborne bacteria, too.

But even without a diffuser, there are other ways to achieve a similar effect. For example, you can use a humidifier by simply adding a few drops of essential oils into it before using. Another method is to pour boiling water into an oven-safe glass bowl and add a few drops of essential oil to it, allowing its aroma to rise with the steam and fill the air until the water temperature cools.

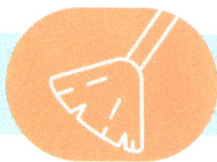

You can also saturate a cotton ball or small cloth with several drops of essential oils and stash it behind a heater or radiator. Or, you can add a couple of drops of an essential oil to the logs in your fireplace to release scent into the room when you light a fire. Some good oils to try are cedarwood, pine, cypress, or fir. Only use a drop or two per log.

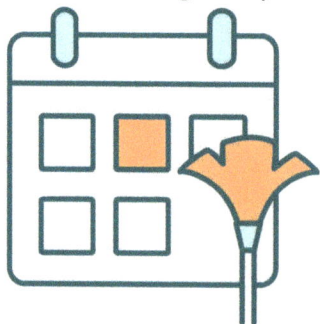

The easiest and least expensive way to use essential oils in the home is to create your own aromatherapy misters. Add 8 to 10 drops of an essential oil or essential oil blend for every 2 ½ cups (or 20 ounces) of water and place in a plant sprayer bottle. Shake thoroughly and use it to spray the air, furnishings, and even the walls on a regular basis to keep them smelling clean and fresh.

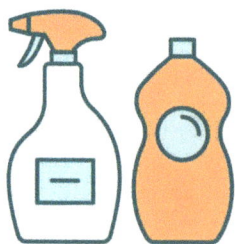

Diffuse essential oils of lemon, lavender, or geranium in bedrooms and hallways to brighten them up. Hallways are often neglected spaces where odors can collect and linger, and benefit most from light, pleasing scents, rather than

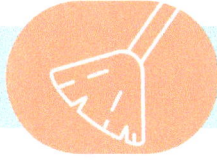

the heavier woodsy or spicy scents more commonly associated with the kitchen or dining areas.

Cleaning Tip: *A Diffuser in the Kitchen*

The kitchen is an ideal spot for a nebulizing diffuser – one that can diffuse oils that effectively to kill odor-causing airborne bacteria and quickly neutralize the heavy odors that linger after cooking, especially after you sauté or fry.

Using Essential Oils for Cleaning Surfaces

All essential oils are antibacterial to some extent, but some also have antiviral and antifungal properties. These will be the best choices to use for cleaning. Not only will they outperform their chemical and synthetic counterparts, but in the long run, they will also be safer and more pleasant for you and everyone in your home.

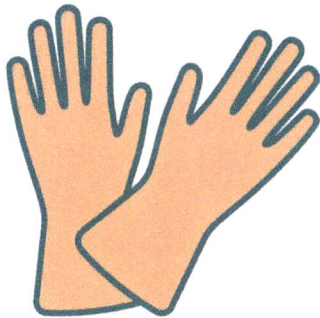

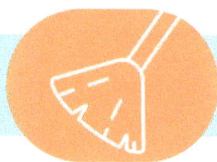

Essential oils that have these properties include lemon, eucalyptus, pine, clove, juniper, rosemary, thyme, oregano, and tea tree. Many of these oils has the added benefit of acting as insect repellents, keeping your home free of unwanted pests.

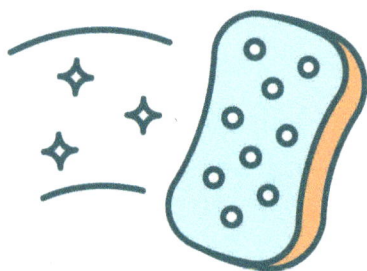

Citrus essential oils leave a clean, fresh scent that is not as overpowering as some of the oils extracted from herbs, and are also useful for cutting through grease. Combine 15 to 20 drops of your favorite oils with ½ cup of distilled white vinegar and 1 ½ cups of water for a general purpose cleaner you can use on counters, floors, cabinets and even windows. For small areas, apply 2 to 3 drops of an individual essential oil or essential oil blend directly to a damp cloth. When using citrus oils, be careful not to apply them directly to appliances as they can damage plastic surfaces.

Using Essential Oils for Deodorizing Carpets and Drapes

An easy way to deodorize rugs and carpets is to make your

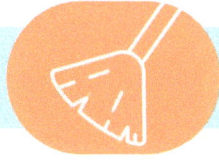

own carpet powder by combining baking soda with a couple of drops of essential oil (the proper ratio is 16 to 20 drops of essential oil per cup of powder). Sprinkle liberally and let it sit for about 10 minutes, then use a vacuum to clean it up.

For drapes, you can use the aromatherapy mister technique. Or you can add a cotton ball or small cloth saturated with essential oils to the collection bag of your vacuum cleaner and use as normal. This will diffuse a pleasant scent while you clean!

Using Essential Oils in the Laundry

The laundry is one of the best and simplest ways you can use essential oils to freshen up and brighten your clothes, towels, and linens. Just add 5 to 10 drops to your laundry detergent or directly to the water for a light scent. To disinfect the laundry, use up to 25 drops of eucalyptus (which has been shown to kill dust mites) or a general purpose, disinfecting blend.

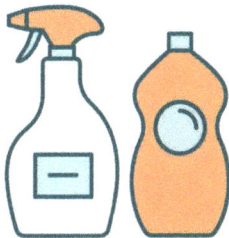

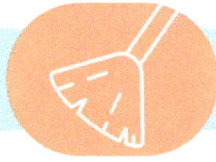

When drying laundry, simply apply 5 to 7 drops of an essential oil or an essential oil blend to a small washcloth and toss it in with your load. You can also make your own laundry sachets with large press 'n brew tea bags. Fill them with herbs such as lavender buds, chamomile flowers, or other fragrant favorites. Or, try your hand at making dryer sheets by adding a couple of drops of a similar or complementary essential oil. You can also use these sachets in your drawers to keep lingerie, socks, and linens smelling fresh.

For bedding, use an essential oil blend that includes chamomile, lavender, marjoram, neroli, or petitgrain on sheets for a scent that promotes restful sleep.

For stains on fabrics or perspiration rings around collars, combine ¼ cup of vinegar with four drops of lemon or eucalyptus essential oil and one tablespoon of baking soda. Rub into stains with an old toothbrush and launder as usual.

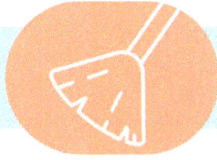

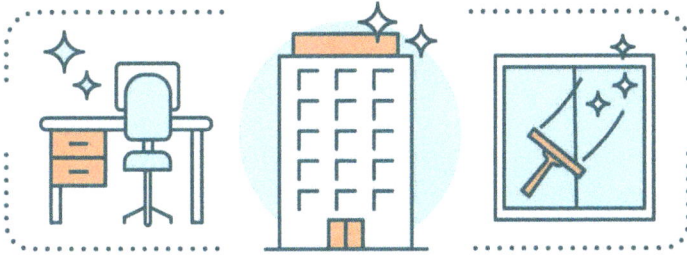

Remove Permanent Marker Stains

You can use lemon essential oil to remove permanent marker stains from many surfaces! Just place a drop of lemon oil on the marker stain, then use a cloth to rub the mark away. Don't be afraid to use a bit of elbow grease!

Streak-Free Mirrors

Add ten drops of lemon essential oil to ¼ cup of vinegar and water and wipe the glass and mirrors clean.

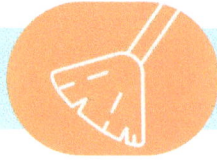

Hand Washing Dishes

Don't have time to make a cleaning product? Try adding several drops of an essential oil such as peppermint, lemon, or pine to your dishwashing liquid.

Sanitize Your Dishwasher

Lemon oil can help dissolve grease and gunk buildup that may be lurking inside your dishwasher. Just add a couple of drops of lemon oil to your dishwasher detergent and run a load as usual!

Eliminate Odors

Lavender essential oil is great for eliminating odors in the air or in fabrics. Make a simple freshening spray by filling an 8-ounce spray bottle with distilled water and 10 to 20 drops of lavender oil. Spritz into the air or onto fabric for instant freshness.

Freshen Carpets

Use essential oils to freshen up musty carpets! In a small bowl, mix one cup of baking soda with ten drops of lemon,

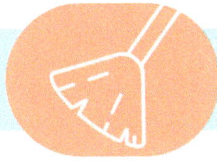

lavender, or peppermint essential oil (or mix and match if you like!) and store in a glass jar with a lid. Sprinkle the baking soda mixture over your carpet the next day; let stand for a half-hour, then vacuum the area thoroughly. Lavender is especially nice to use in a bedroom and more stimulating oils such as lemon or peppermint in living spaces.

Remove Fridge Odors

Strong food smells can permeate your fridge and seep into other foods. Lemon essential oil can take care of unpleasant fridge odors in a snap! Just place three drops of lemon oil onto a sponge and set the sponge in your fridge until the smell is gone.

Deter Pests

Most insects and rodents hate the smell of peppermint essential oil, which makes it a great natural deterrent. Place a few drops of peppermint oil onto a cotton ball and place it inside your cabinets to keep pests at bay. It can be used in the bathroom, kitchen, and around the woodwork in other rooms.

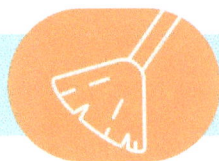

Deodorize Smelly Shoes

Have a pair of smelly sneakers? Use rosemary and lemon essential oil to tame those unpleasant odors! Place five drops of each oil on two cotton balls and put them into the offending shoes. Let them sit overnight, and the shoes will smell much fresher in the morning.

Remove Paint Scent

Adding a fresh coat of paint to any room can make things brighter, but the smell can be overwhelming. To prevent this, stir in one 5ml bottle of your favorite essential oil to any five-gallon bucket of paint.

Remove Sticky Gum or Scuff Marks

If you have a sticky spot or stuck-on gum or glue, try using lemongrass essential oil. Just dab lightly with a couple of drops on a soft cloth and rub off. You can also use lemongrass oil to remove scuff marks on wood floors.

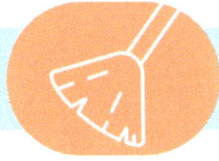

Scrub Away Soap Scum

Tea tree oil can make short work of soap scum in your tub or shower. Just sprinkle some baking soda onto a damp sponge and add a few drops of tea tree oil. Give your tub or shower a scrub and watch the soap scum disappear!

Remove Stains in Fabrics

Got stains? Lemon essential oil can help with them. Add several drops to the washing machine to brighten fabrics and remove tough stains. Or, add a drop to the stained fabric directly before throwing in the wash.

Shine Faucets and Sink

Apply lemon essential oil to a cleaning cloth and rub on chrome faucets and handles to add shine. It works well to remove hard water stains and soap scum on surfaces.

Sanitize Cutting Boards

Soak cutting boards in a solution of two cups of water and 15 drops of lemon essential oil. Wash off afterwards with mild soap and hot water.

Deodorize with Pine

Try using pine essential oil for removing bad odors and freshening up your living areas. It can be used in all kinds of cleaning products for mopping floors, wiping down walls, vacuuming, and much more. Tea tree essential oil also works well as an all-purpose cleaning solution.

Cleaning Tip: *Use Glass*

When making essential oil cleaners, store them in glass whenever possible. Many essential oils can degrade plastic bottles and containers (when not diluted).

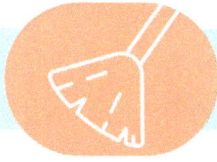

HOW TO CLEAN YOUR HOUSE IN AN HOUR

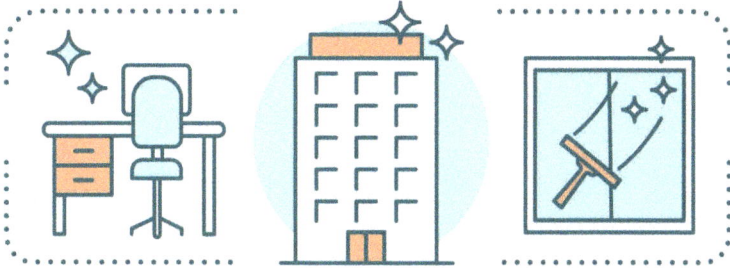

Use this quick checklist to help you get your house clean in just one hour. Professionals have a set schedule and routine for getting it done fast – you can too! Get a boost of motivation by listening to your favorite music or an audio book to distract you from your least favorite chores. And don't forget to dress comfortably and wear comfortable shoes. All those extra steps will go toward your daily goal on your fitness tracker – so multitask away and make those movements count!

Start at the Top

No matter what room you start in, always clean from the

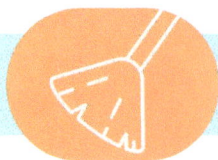

top down, so that dust and dirt fall on lower surfaces that haven't yet been cleaned. For instance, use a duster to clean ceiling fans, then dust furniture (excess dirt will fall to the floor). As your last step, clean all of the floors.

Bedrooms - 5 Minutes Per Room

- Strip the bedsheets and remake the beds with fresh linens. Having an extra set of sheets on hand will save you from having to do laundry right away and return to make the bed.
- Carry an empty basket for clearing all clutter that doesn't belong in that room. Sort through the basket later for organization and return items to their proper place.
- Wipe down bedroom dressers and chests with a dusting spray and cotton cloth, working top to bottom.

Bathrooms - 10 Minutes Per Bath

- Carry all cleaning supplies in a caddy so you can move from one bathroom to the next.
- Clear counters and wipe with sanitizing spray. Clean tub with soft scrub cleaner or spray cleaner and al-

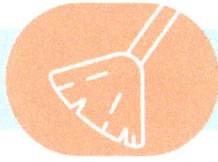

low to sit while you scrub the toilet, then wipe toilet surface and handle.

- Rinse tub and clean mirrors.
- Sweep floor and use a wet mop to clean the floors.

Living and Dining Rooms - 5 Minutes Per Room

- Collect all the clutter that doesn't belong in these rooms and place in the basket.
- Dust ceiling fans and blinds first. Next, dust table-tops and other hard surfaces.
- Clean glass tables and mirrors with spray cleaner.
- Use an upholstery attachment to vacuum uphol-stered furniture. Fold blankets and fluff pillows.
- Sweep hardwood and tile floors and vacuum all car-peting as the final cleaning step.

Kitchen - 10 Minutes

- Load dishwasher with all dirty dishes. Fill the sink with hot soapy water. If your stovetop has remov-able burner pieces that need cleaning, place in wa-ter to soak.
- Remove items from kitchen counters.

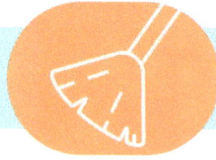

- Dunk sponge in hot soapy water, squeezing out excess and wipe down cabinets, counters and other surfaces, working top to bottom. Rinse the sponge in hot water and repeat until finished. If the countertop is made of granite, use a select wipe or polish as the final step.
- Wipe down appliances.
- Clean any stove knobs or burner pieces and replace.
- Sweep and mop floor last.

Floors - 10 Minutes Entire House

- Start in the furthermost corner of a room, vacuum carpeted rooms, and work your way backward out of the room, moving quickly. Use an attachment to get dust from behind furniture and in corners where pet hair accumulates.
- Swifter mops (reuse the container with your own cleaning solution) or microfiber cloth floor mops make cleaning hard surfaces much faster than traditional mops. Be sure to have a few of these on hand to make your cleaning go more quickly!

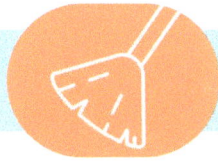

ROOM BY ROOM CLEANING RECIPES

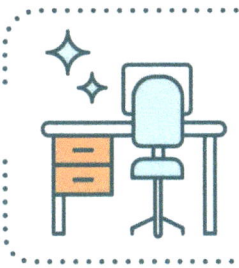

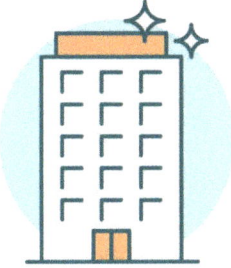

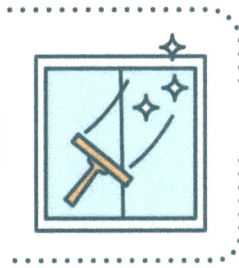

Now, it is time to make your own cleaning supplies. While there are lots of recipes to choose from, the pros say you should be able to tote all of the products you need in one storage caddy, along with all the tools you need – brushes, rags, and trash bags.

There are four basic cleaners you should always have on hand: an abrasive powder cleanser, a tile and bathroom cleaner, a heavy-duty degreaser cleaner, and a light-duty multi-surface cleaner (which doubles as a glass cleaner). These four can usually handle any

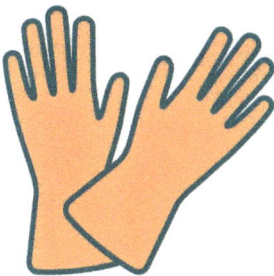

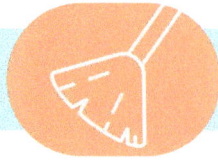

ordinary cleaning chore. But, if those don't do everything you need, there are plenty of other recipes to try! Feel free to tweak any of the recipes by adding a smidgen of this or a tad of that and substitute the suggested essential oils with your favorites.

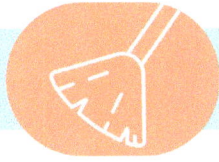

Kitchen

The kitchen is one of the busiest rooms with the most traffic. For some, it is considered the heart of the home where family members gather, share a meal, or celebrate a holiday with friends. For this reason, it is vulnerable to all kinds of bacteria and mold that can creep into nooks and crannies. Essential oils for cleaning in the kitchen include, but are not limited to, lemon, tea tree, lavender, peppermint and orange essential oils.

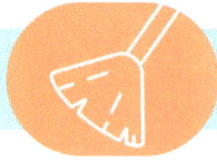

All-Purpose Cleaner with Lemon

What You Will Need:
2 cups white vinegar
2 cups water
1 teaspoon natural dish soap (not castile soap)
30 drops lemon essential oil
20 drops tea tree essential oil
quart-sized spray bottle

What To Do:

1. In a quart-sized spray bottle, add all of the ingredients. Shake to blend.
2. To use, spray and wipe down counters, cabinets, sinks, toilets, and anywhere else needed.

- *Optional:* As an antiseptic or antibacterial disinfectant spray, use eucalyptus, rosemary, or thyme essential oils instead.

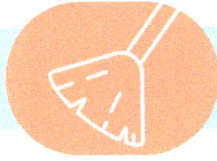

Simple Citrus Soft Scrub

What You Will Need:
1 cup baking soda
¼ cup liquid castile soap
10 drops lemon essential oil
10 drops lime essential oil
10 drops orange essential oil
glass container with lid

What To Do:

1. In a glass container, mix all of the ingredients together to form a paste (add more castile soap if needed).
2. To use, apply with a rag or sponge on stovetop, sinks, or bathtub. Rinse off with clean water.

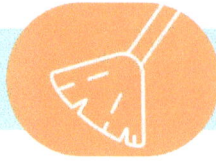

Garbage Disposal Cleaning Bombs

What You Will Need:
2 cups baking soda
1 cup salt
½ cup water
¼ cup liquid castile soap
15 drops orange essential oil
15 drops peppermint essential oil

What To Do:
1. In a bowl, combine baking soda and salt and mix. Add soap and essential oils into mixture and blend.
2. Slowly add water to the mix while stirring, until it has the consistency of damp sand. You will want the mixture to stay together when pressed. Too wet? Add more baking soda. Too dry? Add more water. Do this until the consistency is correct.
3. Form the mixture into balls using hands or a tablespoon and then place on wax paper.
4. Let balls dry until hardened, which usually takes 24 hours.
5. Store in a large, recycled glass container.
6. To use, add one to your garbage disposal when it needs cleaning. Just place one bomb into the disposal, turn on water, and then turn on disposal to run through.

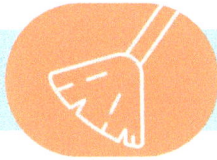

Refrigerator & Microwave Cleaner

What You Will Need:
¼ cup white vinegar
¾ cup hot water
5 drops lemon essential oil
8-ounce glass spray bottle

What To Do:
1. In a glass spray bottle, combine all of the ingredients. Shake well.
2. Spray mixture inside fridge or microwave, then wipe away using a damp cloth.

Alternative method for microwave cleaning:
Heat a cup of water in a microwave-safe container with three drops of lemon essential oil for four minutes or until the point of steaming. Let sit for about five minutes, and then remove the cup. Caution: WATER WILL BE HOT. Wipe down the microwave with a clean cloth.

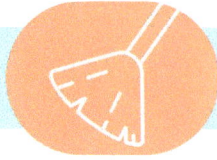

Grease & Grime Remover

What You Will Need:
¼ cup baking soda
4 drops lemon essential oil
1 cup white vinegar
8-ounce glass spray bottle
paper towels

What To Do:

1. Place one cup of vinegar into a glass spray bottle, then set aside.

2. In an empty spice shaker, mix the lemon essential oil and baking soda; set aside.

3. To use, spray the grime buildup with the vinegar spray and then sprinkle essential oil baking soda mixture onto the area.

4. Spray areas again with vinegar spray and allow bubbling reaction to occur. Let sit for 15 minutes.

5. Finally, wipe clean with paper towels to remove grease and grime. Repeat if needed for any stubborn areas.

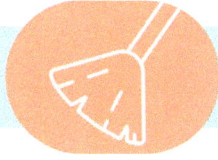

Natural Stovetop Cleaner

What You Will Need:
¼ cup baking soda
¼ cup salt
1 tablespoon white vinegar
2 tablespoons water
5 drops lime essential oil

What To Do:
1. In a small container, stir in all of the ingredients until they form a paste.
2. Spread mixture over the stovetop and burner rings. Leave it on for 15 minutes, or longer for tough stains.
3. Using a sponge, scrub mixture into the grime. Remove gunk and wipe surface clean.

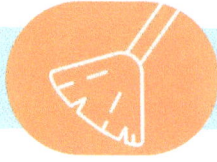

Stainless Steel Appliance Spray

What You Will Need:
2 drops lavender essential oil
2 drops lemon essential oil
½ cup fractionated coconut oil
2-ounce spray bottle

What To Do:
1. In a spray bottle, combine all of the ingredients. Shake well before using.
2. To use on an appliance, spray cleaner on the surface and rub in to polish surface with a soft, clean cloth.

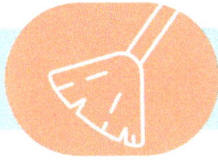

Microwave Sparkle Cleaner

Does your microwave still smell like the popcorn you made in it a week ago? Sometimes food odors get trapped inside the microwave, along with grease, spills, and splatters. Here's an easy way to take care of your oven and keep it clean.

What You Will Need:
5-6 drops lemon essential oil
¼ cup baking soda
1 teaspoon vinegar
bowl
sponge

What To Do:

1. Mix baking soda, vinegar and essential oil in a bowl.
2. Use a sponge or clean cloth to apply the paste and lightly scrub your microwave.
3. Rinse the sponge and wipe clean.

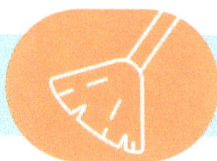

Natural Scouring Powder

What You Will Need:
2 cups baking soda
8 drops tea tree essential oil
8 drops lemon essential oil
2 tablespoons rosemary leaves (ground)
Shaker bottle with lid

What To Do:

1. Grind the rosemary leaves and set aside. In a separate bowl, add essential oils to the baking soda. Stir in rosemary leaves and mix well.

2. Place mixture in a shaker bottle and replace the lid. Use as needed.

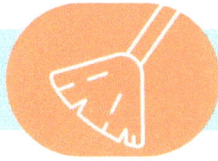

Creamy Soft Scrub

What You Will Need:
4 cups baking soda
1 cup castile liquid soap
½ cup vegetable glycerin soap
10 drops tea tree essential oil
aluminum canister with lid

What To Do:
1. In a bowl, add all liquid ingredients together and stir. Add baking soda in last.
2. Place scrub in the aluminum canister.
3. Use this scrub for cleaning stoves, countertops, bathrooms, and sinks.

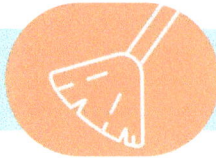

Lime Essential Oil Soft Scrub

What You Will Need:
½ cup baking soda
2 tablespoons castile soap
1 tablespoon water
10 drops lime essential oil
glass container with lid

What To Do:
1. In a bowl, add all of the ingredients and mix well.
2. Use on stovetop, sinks, tub, etc.
3. Store any leftover mixture in a glass container with other cleaning products.

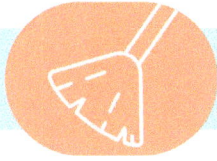

All-Purpose Surface Cleaner with Lavender

What You Will Need:
¾ cups distilled water
2 tablespoons white vinegar
15 drops lavender essential oil
15 drops orange essential oil
8-ounce spray bottle

What To Do:
1. Combine all of the ingredients in a spray bottle and shake well.
2. Before use, shake well. Spray on surface area and wipe clean.

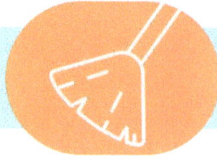

Pine Floor Cleaner

What You Will Need:
1 gallon of water
2 tablespoons castile soap
15 drops white fir essential oil
5 drops lemon essential oil
mop and bucket

What To Do:

1. Place all of the ingredients into mop bucket or use the kitchen sink with a closed drain. Stir well.
2. Mop, as usual, using the cleaning solution on floors. No need to rinse off. Allow the floor to air dry.

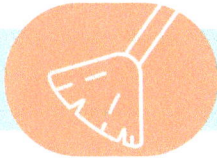

Pine Floor Cleaner #2

This one is just like the pine floor cleaners from the store, except it's all-natural, which means it is healthy for you and your pets.

What You Will Need:

10 drops pine essential oil
5 drops tea tree essential oil
5 drops cypress essential oil
2 tablespoons liquid castile soap
1 gallon water
bucket

What To Do:

1. Fill the bucket with hot water, then add essential oils and soap.
2. Mix well and mop as usual.
3. Rinsing is not necessary, and you will be delighted with the pine fragrance on your tile floors.

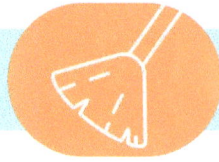

Kitchen Floor Cleaner

Looking for a natural way to scrub those tough stains? Here's a great home remedy for fighting grease. Give this vinegar formula a try.

What You Will Need:

20 drops tea tree essential oil
2 tablespoons liquid castile soap
¼ baking soda
1 cup vinegar
1 gallon water

What To Do:

1. Fill a clean bucket with water. Add all of the ingredients, mixing well.
2. Clean your floor as usual. Rinsing is not necessary.
3. For stubborn stains, drop essential oil directly on the spot and wait a few minutes, then scrub off.

- *Recipe variation:* Substitute the tea tree oil for 20 drops of peppermint essential oil, 20 drops of eucalyptus essential oil, or 15 drops of orange essential oil and 5 drops of lemon essential oil.

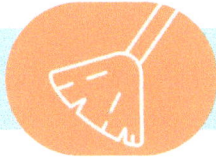

Window Spray Cleaner

What You Will Need:
3 tablespoons white vinegar
1 teaspoon rubbing alcohol
10 drops citrus oil of choice
3/4 cup water
8-ounce glass spray bottle

What To Do:

1. Combine all ingredients except for water in glass bottle, swirl to mix. Fill the rest of bottle with water.

2. Replace spray top and shake well to blend.

3. For best results, use with a microfiber cloth.

- *Note:* Rubbing alcohol is the secret ingredient to preventing streaks; however, it can be omitted if not desired.

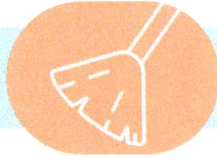

Kitchen Citrus Soap Wedges

These little soap wedges will brighten your kitchen with color and zest.

What You Will Need:
½ pound transparent melt and pour base
½ tablespoon coconut oil
3 drops lemon essential oil
3 drops grapefruit essential oil
3 drops orange essential oil
soap mold (fruit wedges)
orange, yellow, and green food coloring

What To Do:
1. Melt the soap base and coconut oil in the microwave in a glass container.
2. Add essential oils and mix well. Using another bowl or container, divide the soap base, and add the appropriate food color, then pour into the fruit wedge mold.

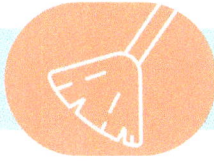

Appliance Cleaner

Here's an easy recipe that works as a degreaser and will make your appliances sparkle.

What You Will Need:

10 drops rosemary essential oil
¼ cup oil-based soap (i.e., Murphy's)
2 cups water
spray bottle

What To Do:

1. Combine all ingredients in a clean spray bottle.
2. Shake well before using. Spray generously on appliances and let sit a few minutes. Wipe clean as usual.

*   *Recipe variation:* Use ten drops of lavender essential oil or lemon essential oil in place of rosemary essential oil.

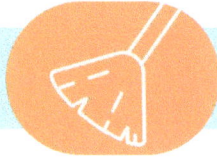

Appliance Cleaner #2

Here's another cleaner that's especially great for stovetops and refrigerators.

What You Will Need:

4 drops lemon essential oil
1 teaspoon liquid castile soap
1 teaspoon borax
¼ cup lemon juice
1/8 cup white vinegar
2 cups water
spray bottle

What To Do:

1. Combine all ingredients in a clean spray bottle.
2. Shake bottle to mix well. Spray generously on appliance surface then wipe off with a damp sponge. Wipe surface again using a clean cloth.

- *Recipe variation:* Use four drops of orange essential oil or eucalyptus essential oil in place of lemon essential oil.

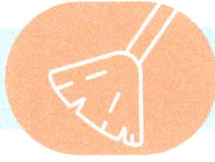

Homemade Citrus Dish Soap

What You Will Need:
3/4 cup liquid castile soap
2 teaspoons vegetable glycerin
1 ½ teaspoons baking soda
10 drops lemon essential oil
5 drops orange essential oil
5 drops tea tree essential oil
8-ounce glass bottle with pump top

What To Do:
1. In a glass bowl, gently whisk all of the ingredients until blended together.
2. Using a funnel, pour into the spray bottle.
3. To use, add a few squirts to dish water as the sink is filling or place a small amount on a washcloth to hand wash dishes.

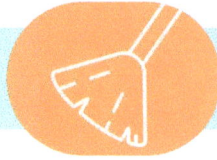

All-Natural Disinfecting Spray

What You Will Need:
3 tablespoons white vinegar
10 drops peppermint essential oil
10 drops orange essential oil
10 drops eucalyptus essential oil
¾ cup water
8-ounce spray bottle

What To Do:

1. In a spray bottle, add water, white vinegar, and essential oils. Replace spray top and shake to blend.

2. To use, spray on countertops, stovetops, and other surfaces to disinfect. Wipe surface dry.

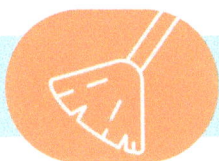

Kitchen Sink Scrub

Use this cleaner in place of other harsh brands to scrub sinks.

What You Will Need:
1 cup baking soda
¼ cup vinegar
10 drops lemon essential oil
10 drops orange essential oil
bowl

What To Do:
1. Combine all ingredients in a small bowl. Mix well.
2. Use as a kitchen sink and tub scrub.

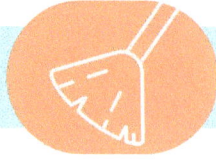

Citrus Glass Cleaner

Use this homemade spray to clean glass and polish mirrors. It will add a wonderful, refreshing fragrance in every room.

What You Will Need:

4 ounces water
4 ounces apple cider vinegar
1 tablespoon borax
1 tablespoon orange essential oil
1 tablespoon lemon essential oil
spray bottle

What To Do:

1. Combine all ingredients in a spray bottle and shake well.
2. Spray on surfaces and wipe immediately. Shake before each use.

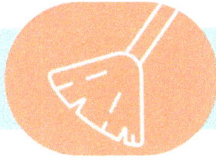

Refrigerator Cleaner

Sometimes a box of baking soda isn't enough to keep your refrigerator or freezer smelling fresh. Here's an easy recipe for a cleaner that will make it sparkle.

What You Will Need:
10 drops peppermint essential oil
3 tablespoons baking soda
½ cup water

What To Do:

1. In a bowl, mix water, essential oil and baking soda.
2. Clean as usual, wiping down shelves and door.

- *Recipe variation:* Use eucalyptus essential oil for cleaning the freezer.

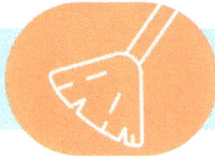

Glass & Surface Cleaner

What You Will Need:
1 cup white vinegar
1 cup water
¼ cup rubbing alcohol
10 drops rosemary essential oil
10 drops lemon essential oil
5 drops peppermint essential oil
spray bottle

What To Do:

1. Mix all ingredients in a spray bottle.
2. Shake well before each use and use as normal to clean glass tables, mirrors, and countertops.

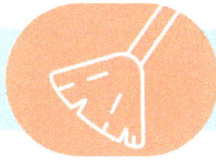

Dishwashing Liquid Soap

This soap is for hand washing your dishes. While it sanitizes your dishes, it will lift your spirit and strengthen your nails all at the same time.

What You Will Need:
16 ounces liquid castile soap (or mild dishwashing liquid)
10 drops orange essential oil
10 drops lemon essential oil
10 drops lavender essential oil
squirt bottle

What To Do:

1. Combine all of the ingredients into a squirt bottle. Shake well.
2. Use as normal for hand washing your dishes.

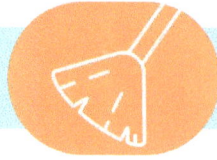

Dishwasher Detergent Powder

To add fragrance, improve the antiseptic action, and help disinfect dishes, add several drops of essential oils such as lavender, tea tree, fir, spruce, pine, lemon, bergamot, or orange.

What You Will Need:

2 cups borax
2 cups washing soda
1 cup citric acid
1 cup salt
20 drops grapefruit essential oil (or substitute: lavender)

What To Do:

1. Combine all ingredients and store in an airtight container.
2. Use one tablespoon per load as needed.
3. For an extra boost, add a few drops of dishwashing liquid to the powder when adding to the dishwasher.
4. Add white vinegar as the rinse agent.

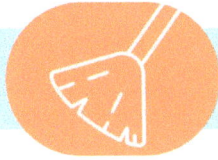

Kitchen Mop & Glow

Degrease your kitchen with citrus essential oils that make your kitchen smell great, too.

What You Will Need:
8 drops lemon essential oil
15 drops orange essential oil
2 tablespoons liquid castile soap
1 gallon water
bucket

What To Do:
1. Fill the bucket with hot water.
2. Add essential oils and soap.
3. Mix well.
4. Mop or scrub floor as usual. No rinsing necessary.

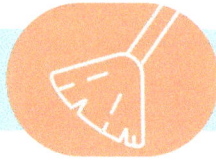

Heavy-Duty Overnight Oven Cleaner

This recipe is proven to do the heavy work for you while you sleep!

What You Will Need:
1 ½ cups baking soda
1 cup water
½ cup salt
¼ cup vinegar
2 teaspoons liquid castile soap
10 drops lemon or orange essential oil

What To Do:
1. Preheat oven at 300 degrees for 15 minutes. Turn off oven and open door.
2. In a plastic bottle, add water and essential oil. Shake well.
3. Spray on the bottom of the oven and sides.
4. Combine ¼ cup of salt and ½ cup of baking soda and sprinkle on the oven floor and over spilled areas.
5. Mix ¼ cup of water, ¾ cup of baking soda, ¼ cup of salt, and castile soap. Again, cover the walls of the oven with this mixture. Allow to sit overnight.
6. In the morning, add ½ cup of water and vinegar in the spray bottle and spray on the wall and bottom of

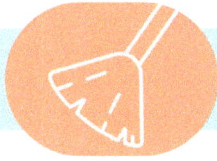

the oven into the mixture. Wipe off, using steel wool to hit baked on spots. Rinse several times to remove all residue.

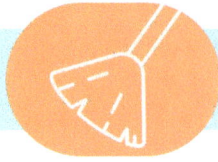

Swifty Floor Wipes

If you use convenient electrostatic floor cleaners with disposal wipes, you can make your own using cellulose cloth cut into rectangles.

What You Will Need:
1 cup water
1 cup vinegar
10 drops lemon essential oil (or substitute: rosemary)
10 drops geranium essential oil
bowl
pre-cut cellulose cloths
Ziploc bag

What To Do:
1. In a bowl, add all of the ingredients and stir well.
2. Place the cloths in the mixture and allow the wipes to soak up the liquid.
3. Transfer the cloths into a plastic Ziploc bag. Add ¼ cup of liquid to keep moist during storage.
4. Use your homemade floor wipes on tile, linoleum, or wood floors.

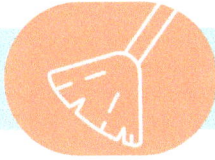

Fruit & Veggie Cleaning Spray

Before taking a bite, be sure to wash your fruit and vegetables from the grocery store.

What You Will Need:
½ cup water
2 drops grapefruit essential oil
2 drops lemon essential oil
½ teaspoon baking soda
4-ounce spray bottle

What To Do:

1. Add all of your ingredients into a spray bottle. Replace sprayer and shake to blend well.
2. Spray fruits and vegetables in a colander, then rinse with cool running water. Let air dry.

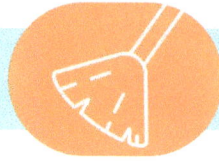

Bathroom

Cleaning in the bathroom requires strong essential oils, such as peppermint, eucalyptus, or tea tree. Since skin and hair sheds and can attract tiny insects, spraying your bathroom with peppermint essential oil after it has been cleaned is a great way to keep your bathroom sanitized and detract any pests. Spray around the bottom of the toilet and faucet, under the sink and edges of the floor, and inside the wastebasket. Tea tree oil will remove mold and mildew. Vinegar is your best friend for mirrors and polishing faucets.

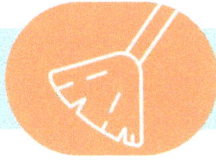

Shower Head Cleaner

What You Will Need:
white vinegar
5 drops lemon essential oil
gallon-sized ziploc bag

What To Do:

1. Remove shower head and place into a ziploc bag.

2. Add vinegar and lemon essential oil to bag, seal and let soak for several hours.

3. Alternatively, if you are unable to remove the shower head, you can place the vinegar and oil in the ziploc bag and then place the bag over the shower head and use a rubber band to hold in place while it soaks.

- *Note:* Be sure to not overfill the bag; use just enough to cover the head to remove mineral deposits.

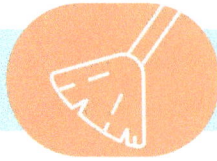

Mold & Mildew Cleaner

What You Will Need:
5 drops tea tree essential oil
5 drops lavender essential oil
5 drops orange essential oil
5 drops thyme essential oil
5 drops oregano essential oil
1 teaspoon borax
2/3 cup white vinegar
¼ cup distilled water
8-ounce glass bottle with sprayer

What To Do:
1. In a glass bowl, combine all of the ingredients and whisk until well blended.
2. Pour into the spray bottle using a funnel. Shake well before use.
3. To use, spray on problem areas and let sit for 15 minutes. Wipe clean with a damp microfiber cloth.

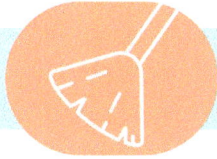

Lavender Foaming Hand Soap

What You Will Need:
2 tablespoons castile soap
15 drops lavender essential oil
2 teaspoons olive oil
1 cup distilled water
10-ounce foaming soap pump

What To Do:
1. In a foaming soap bottle, add soap, essential oils and olive oil. Swirl to gently mix together.
2. Add water to bottle and replace pump top on bottle. Shake well to mix.
3. To use, pump twice into palm of hand and lather well, rinse off and dry hands.

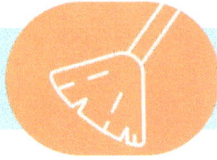

Tea Tree Toilet Cleaner

What You Will Need:
1 cup white vinegar
1 cup baking soda
¼ cup salt
10 drops tea tree essential oil
glass container with shaker lid
spray bottle

What To Do:

1. In a container with a shaker lid, add the baking soda, salt, and tea tree oil and mix.
2. In a spray bottle, add the vinegar and set aside.
3. To use, spray the vinegar in the toilet bowl, then sprinkle in the powder mix. Let the fizz reaction occur, and spray more vinegar if needed.
4. Let sit for 15 minutes, then scrub with a toilet brush. Flush when finished.

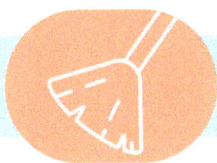

Tea Tree Cleaning Wipes

What You Will Need:

1 roll premium paper towels
2 cups warm distilled water
15 drops tea tree essential oil
1 tablespoon castile soap
container with airtight lid or gallon ziploc bag

What To Do:

1. Cut paper towel roll in half with a serrated knife, using half now and saving the other half for a second batch.

2. Combine water, essential oil, and castile soap in a small bowl. Place paper towel roll into container with lid or ziploc bag.

3. Pour mixture over paper towels and allow it to soak in for ten minutes.

4. Turn the container or ziploc bag over and let sit for another ten minutes.

5. Remove cardboard tube from paper towels and discard. Pull the wipes from center of the roll to use. Keep container covered or sealed when not in use.

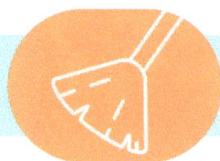

Soft Lavender Scrub

Lavender makes this cleaner a joy to use.

What You Will Need:

¾ cup baking soda
¼ cup powdered milk
1/8 cup liquid castile soap
5 drops lavender essential oil
water
squeeze bottle

What To Do:

1. Combine baking soda, milk, castile soap and lavender in a squeeze bottle.
2. Add water to create a smooth paste. Shake to mix. Apply to the surface, then wipe with a damp sponge to clean.

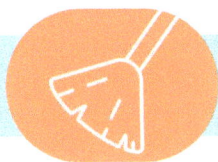

Tub & Shower Gel

What You Will Need:
1 cup white vinegar
½ cup natural dishwashing liquid (not castile soap)
10 drops lavender essential oil
squeeze bottle

What To Do:
1. In a small saucepan, heat the vinegar on the stove-top until hot (but not boiling).
2. Carefully stir in the dishwashing soap until blended.
3. Remove from heat and allow to cool. Stir in the essential oil, and then pour into the squeeze bottle.
4. To use, squirt into tub and shower and allow to sit for one hour. Wipe off with a moist sponge. Rinse and repeat.

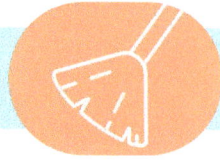

Peppermint Daily Shower Spray

What You Will Need:
¼ cup vodka (or rubbing alcohol if preferred)
¾ cup water
10 drops peppermint essential oil
8-ounce spray bottle

What To Do:

1. In a spray bottle, combine all of the ingredients. Shake to mix well.

2. To use, shake before use. Spray in shower and on walls every day. No rinse is required.

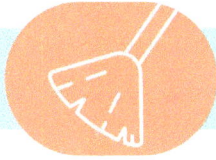

Deep Clean Toilet Scrub

What You Will Need:
½ cup baking soda
1/3 cup liquid dishwashing soap
¼ cup hydrogen peroxide
30 drops eucalyptus essential oil
¾ cup water
squeeze-top bottle

What To Do:

1. Use a funnel to add liquids and dry ingredients into a squeeze-top bottle. Shake to mix.
2. To use, squirt into the toilet under the rim. Scrub, then let stand ten minutes before flushing.

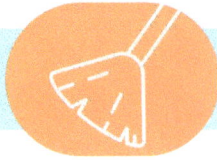

Daily Shower Spray

What You Will Need:
1 ½ cups water
1 cup white vinegar
½ cup rubbing alcohol
1 teaspoon liquid dish soap (not castile soap)
15 drops lime essential oil
15 drops tea tree essential oil
large spray bottle

What To Do:

1. Combine all of the ingredients into a quart-sized spray bottle.

2. Spray daily on shower door and walls after use (this spray is a preventative spray, designed to help prevent build-up).

- *Optional:* Since this bottle will be left in the shower to be used daily, consider getting creative and decorating your spray bottle.

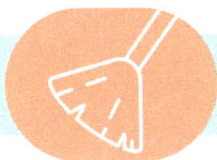

Minty Fresh Window & Mirror Cleaner

What You Will Need:
3 cups distilled water
¼ cup vodka (or rubbing alcohol)
¼ cup vinegar
20 drops peppermint or spearmint essential oil
large spray bottle

What To Do:
1. Combine all of the ingredients in a quart-sized spray bottle. Shake to blend.
2. To use, spray on mirrors, windows, or stainless steel. Wipe off with paper towels or old newspaper for streak-free shine.

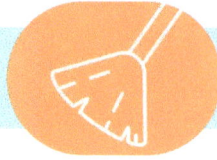

Bathroom Air Freshener

Keep your bathroom clean from viruses and bacteria with this refreshing air spray.

What You Will Need:

5 drops lemon essential oil
5 drops cinnamon essential oil
5 drops eucalyptus essential oil
5 drops sage essential oil
5 drops thyme essential oil
10 drops lavender essential oil
10 drops tea tree essential oil
10 drops rosemary essential oil
distilled water
spray bottle

What To Do:

1. Fill a spray bottle with eight ounces of distilled water, then add essential oils.
2. Shake this mixture well before each use. Spray every day to keep your bathroom smelling fresh and clean.

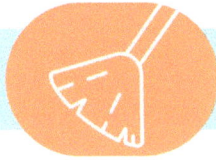

Bathroom Cleaner

What You Will Need:
2-3 drops cinnamon essential oil
2-3 drops eucalyptus essential oil
2-3 drops lemon essential oil
2-3 drops lavender essential oil
2-3 drops tea tree essential oil
distilled water
8-ounce spray bottle

What To Do:

1. Fill a spray bottle with distilled water and add essential oils. If you do not have all of the essential oils listed, you can substitute with another essential oil or double the drops of one. Do not leave tea tree essential oil out, though, as this one is the most beneficial.

2. Shake well before each use. Spray in the shower to keep clean and sparkling. Spray on the toilet seat and wipe down. Use on surfaces and doorknobs to disinfect and sanitize. Your bathroom will look fresh and polished and have a rich, refreshing scent you can only get with pure essential oils.

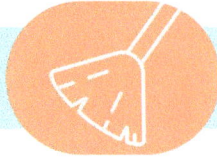

Tub-A-Dub Cleaner

Get rid of that ugly mold and mildew buildup in your bath-room using these essential oils.

What You Will Need:

1 cup baking soda
20 drops tea tree essential oil
20 drops lavender essential oil
20 drops lemon essential oil
bowl

What To Do:

1. In a bowl, combine all ingredients and mix well.

2. Using a damp sponge, scrub tub or shower with cleaner. For tough stains or mildew buildup, leave on for 15 minutes, then scrub.

- *Recipe Variation:* Make your own Fresh Shower Spray by combining essential oils in a spray bottle with water. Spray shower daily after each use.

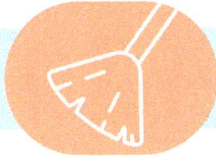

X-Mildew Formula

This formula helps fight fungus, mildew, and mold in your home. Diffuse daily.

What You Will Need:
½ teaspoon tea tree essential oil
½ teaspoon clove bud essential oil
½ teaspoon lavender essential oil
saucepan or diffuser

What To Do:

1. Combine all essential oils in a saucepan of water or diffuser.
2. Use as needed. Diffuse for 10-15 minutes twice a day.

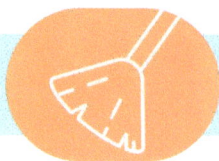

Disinfectant Handy Wipes

Make these in advance to carry with you.

What You Will Need:

15-20 drops essential oil blend
1 cup distilled water
1 roll paper towels (half-sheet size)
casserole dish
bowl
quart-sized plastic Ziploc bag

What To Do:

1. Cut or tear paper towels in half into 20-25 squares. Place towels in the bottom of a casserole dish.

2. Combine water and essential oil blend in a bowl. Mix well.

3. Pour essential oil mixture into the casserole, allowing the towels to absorb the liquid. Lightly ring the excess liquid off then fold in half and place in a plastic Ziploc bag or an empty wipe container. Use as needed.

- *Recipe Variation:* For cleaning little hands, add ¼ cup of natural baby shampoo to your recipe.

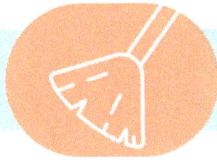

Poo-Poo Spray

This is an all-natural version of the popular toilet spray to use before you flush!

What You Will Need:
2 ounces distilled water
1 drop glycerin (or substitute: castile soap)
1 tablespoon rubbing alcohol (or substitute: vodka or witch hazel)
16 drops essential oils (your choice)
2-ounce spray bottle

What To Do:

1. In a glass spray bottle, add essential oils, glycerin, and rubbing alcohol. Shake to blend.

2. Add water to fill the rest of the bottle. Shake to blend.

3. Leave in bathroom on toilet for family members and visitors to use before using restroom.

- *Note:* Popular essential oil combinations for scents include: bergamot + lemongrass + grapefruit; spearmint + eucalyptus; or lavender + vanilla.

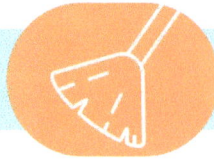

Bedroom

Running a diffuser with a soft floral oil or another delicate-scented essential oil before retiring for the night will help create a relaxing atmosphere. Use a linen spray on bedsheets when making the bed to keep fresh. Or, place a bowl of potpourri on a dresser or nightstand for added fragrance.

If a clothes hamper is close by, add a few drops of essential oils to the lid for keeping dirty laundry smells at bay. For the closet, make a sachet of dried potpourri in a mesh bag. Add several drops of essential oil to it. Hang over a hanger or place in a chest of linens for freshening a closed space. Refresh as needed. Lavender and rose are classic scents for lingerie drawers. For children's sleepwear, roman chamomile is especially fragrant and relaxing.

Refresh your room by spritzing blinds, shades, draperies, and other window treatments with essential oils. Just fill a spray bottle with water and a drop of glycerin, then add your favorite essential oil. Don't forget to add essential oils to your cleaning solution when washing plastic blinds and shutters.

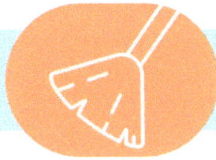

Bed Bug Mattress Spray

What You Will Need:
½ cup vodka
½ cup distilled water
8 drops lavender essential oil
4 drops peppermint essential oil
4 drops tea tree essential oil
4 drops eucalyptus essential oil
8-ounce glass bottle with spray top

What To Do:

1. Combine all of the ingredients into a glass spray bottle and shake to blend.
2. To use, shake to mix ingredients, then spray on mattress and let air dry.

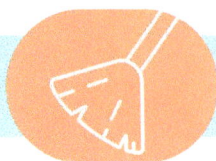

Fresh Linen Spray

What You Will Need:
¼ cup distilled water
3 tablespoons witch hazel or vodka
20 drops lavender essential oil
15 drops frankincense essential oil
Small spray bottle

What To Do:
1. In a small spritzer bottle, add all of the ingredients. Shake well.
2. To use, spray on bedsheets, pillowcases, and linens.

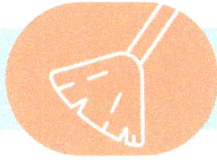

Sweet Fields Air Freshener

What You Will Need:
3/4 cup distilled water
2 tablespoons vodka or rubbing alcohol (optional: real vanilla extract)
10 drops lavender essential oil
5 drops roman chamomile essential oil
8-ounce spray bottle

What To Do:
1. Combine all of the ingredients in an 8-ounce spray bottle. Shake to blend.
2. Spray throughout the house to eliminate odors or stale smells.

- *Note:* Other essential oil combinations to try include orange and cinnamon or mandarin and silver fir.

Cleaning Tip: *Considering that we spend about one-third of our time in our bedroom, this is an important room to make sure the air quality is good for rest.*

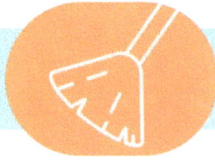

Sickroom Deodorizer Diffuser Blend

What You Will Need:

6 drops rosemary essential oil
6 drops grapefruit essential oil
4 drops lemon essential oil
2 drops eucalyptus essential oil
5ml glass bottle with lid

What To Do:

1. In a small 5ml glass bottle, combine essential oils, replace the cap and shake to blend.

2. Add several drops to a diffuser to combat odors and kill germs during cold and flu season.

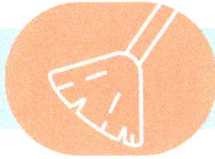

Lavender Perfumed Lining Paper

Find a pretty lining paper and spice it up with a lovely fragrance.

What You Will Need:
lining paper
blotting paper
6 drops lavender essential oil
large plastic bag

What To Do:

1. Cut lining paper to size and place sheets together in a plastic bag.

2. Add several drops of lavender essential oil to blotting paper and place in a plastic bag with lining paper.

3. Leave paper in the bag for a week to absorb the fragrance.

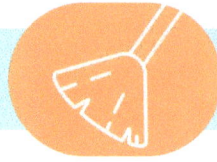

Living Areas

Cleanse the air in your living space with a diffuser and your favorite essential oil. Dust table tops and lamps with a gentle essential oil, such as lavender.

Note: since citrus oils are great for breaking down buildup of products, they will do so on treated table tops. Therefore, it isn't recommended to use citrus essential oils on treated table tops or as a fabric cleanser. You can spray couches and rugs with a gentle cleanser, such as lavender or chamomile, without worrying about a breakdown of fabric or polish.

Olive oil can be used to treat untreated wood. It will give it a nice shine and condition it to prevent cracks.

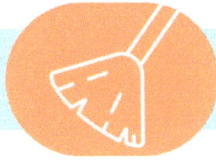

Lemon Furniture Polish

What You Will Need:
½ cup olive oil
40 drops lemon essential oil
½ cup white distilled vinegar
Squeeze-top bottle

What To Do:

1. In a squeeze-top bottle, add all of the ingredients and seal with the cap. Shake to blend.
2. Squeeze polish onto a clean, dry cloth and rub wood in the direction of the grain. Use a soft brush to work the polish into corners or tight places.

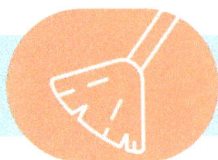

Simple Furniture Polish

What You Will Need:

1/4 cup olive oil
5 drops lemon essential oil
2-ounce glass lotion pump bottle

What To Do:

1. In a glass bottle, add olive oil and essential oil. Shake well.

2. To use, squirt several pumps onto a microfiber cloth and wipe wood surfaces clean.

- *Note:* Polish furniture every other month. Use dusting spray to keep surfaces clean between times with polish. Alternatively, you can wipe down surfaces with a damp microfiber cloth.

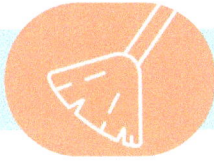

Dusting Spray

What You Will Need:
1 teaspoon olive oil
3 tablespoons white vinegar
10 drops white fir or lemon essential oil
¾ cup distilled water
8-ounce glass spray bottle

What To Do:
1. In a spray bottle, combine all of the ingredients, except water. Swirl to combine.
2. Fill the rest of the bottle with water. Screw on top and shake to mix well.
3. To use, shake and lightly mist onto microfiber cloth. Wipe down surfaces.

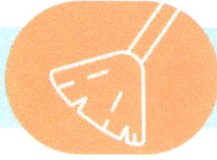

Lemon Carpet Refresher

What You Will Need:
1 cup baking soda
30 drops lemon essential oil
glass container with lid

What To Do:
1. In a small glass container, add baking soda then stir in the essential oil. Cover tightly with a lid. Shake well and allow to sit for 6 to 8 hours.
2. Sprinkle on stale or smelly carpet and allow to sit overnight. Vacuum up the next morning.

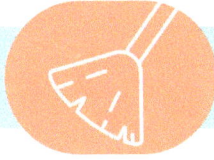

Be Free of Fleas Carpet Treatment

Rid your house of annoying pests. Be sure to repeat regularly to avoid infestation of fleas in the home where pets dwell.

What You Will Need:

1 ¼ cups baking soda
3 drops lemongrass essential oil
10 drops orange essential oil
10 drops citronella essential oil
4 drops peppermint essential oil
plastic container

What To Do:

1. In a container, combine all of the ingredients and mix well.
2. Sprinkle heavily over the entire carpet. Let sit for one hour. Vacuum up and discard the vacuum bag.

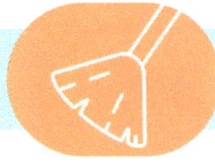

Garden Fresh Carpet Shampoo

What You Will Need:
2 cups baking soda
2 cups water
½ cup soap flakes (or substitute: borax)
½ cup vinegar
20 drops lavender essential oil
8 drops rosemary essential oil

What To Do:

1. Vacuum rug before using this carpet shampoo. In a bowl, combine baking soda and soap flakes (or borax).

2. Add essential oils and stir to blend well. Sprinkle over the carpet.

3. In a bucket, add vinegar and water. Wet sponge mop and go over the carpet working in the baking soda mixture. Continue to rinse mop and go over the entire carpet. Wait an hour before vacuuming the carpet.

- *Note:* The formula can be used in a carpet steamer by reducing or increasing cleaner amounts according to the type of machine you use. Be sure to check colorfastness in an inconspicuous area of carpet before using the formula for the first time.

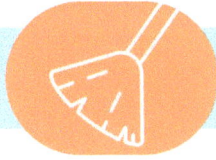

Carpet Steamer Shampoo

Use this formula in a steam-cleaning machine instead of the store-bought shampoos.

What You Will Need:
¾ cup hot water
½ white vinegar
1 tablespoon liquid castile soap
35 drops thyme essential oil

What To Do:

1. Using a container with a pouring spout, add all of the ingredients and blend well.

2. Add the formula into the steaming machine per manufacturer directions and use according to the manufacturer's directions.

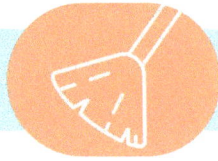

Goo & Crayon Remover

What You Will Need:
10 drops lemon essential oil
1 tablespoons fractionated coconut oil or almond oil (optional)
15ml glass bottle with lid

What To Do:
1. In a small glass 15ml bottle, add the coconut oil and essential oil. Replace reducer and cap and shake to blend.
2. To use, apply directly to the sticker residue, random goo, gum, crayon marks, etc.
3. Rub in with fingers, then wipe away with a clean rag. Repeat as needed.

- *Note:* Be sure to test in an inconspicuous place first if you are worried about the surface becoming discolored or damaged.

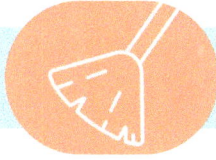

Living Room Freshening Spray

What You Will Need:
5 drops bergamot essential oil
3 drops cinnamon essential oil
1 drop frankincense essential oil
3 drops pine essential oil
¼ teaspoon soft soap
15 ounces water
large spray bottle

What To Do:
1. In a spray bottle, add water, soft soap, and essential oils. Replace trigger sprayer top and shake to blend.
2. To use, spray on countertops and other surfaces to disinfect. Wipe surface dry.

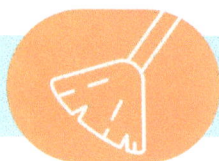

Room Spray

Freshen up your house with fragrant oils.

What You Will Need:

1 ½ ounces distilled water
1 ½ ounces vodka
20 drops rosemary essential oil
4 drops peppermint essential oil
8 drops lemon essential oil
4 drops lavender essential oil
8-ounce spray bottle

What To Do:

1. Fill the spray bottle with distilled water and alcohol (or just 3 ounces of distilled water).
2. Add essential oils. Shake before each use.
3. Mist each room lightly. Be careful to not use on fabric furniture.

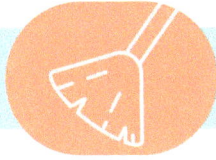

Lavender & Tea Tree Cleaning Spray

What You Will Need:

1 teaspoon borax
2 tablespoons white vinegar
2 cups hot water
20 drops lavender essential oil
5 drops tea tree essential oil
large spray bottle

What To Do:

1. In a large glass spray bottle, add all of the ingredients and essential oils. Replace top and shake until dry ingredients dissolve.
2. Spray on any hard surface (except glass) and scrub with a clean cloth, then rinse.

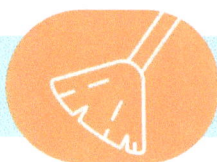

Scented Rocks

Make your own scented rocks to use like potpourri in a dish.

What You Will Need:
½ cup flour
½ cup salt
¼ teaspoon essential oil (any fragrance you like)
½ cup boiling water
food coloring

What To Do:
1. In a bowl, mix the flour and salt.
2. Add the essential oil and boiling water to the dry ingredients.
3. Add food coloring to create the desired color. Blend well.
4. Take a small amount to shape balls in different sizes to make stones. (Add more water if too dry.)
5. Allow to dry, then place in a dish or bowl to scent a room.

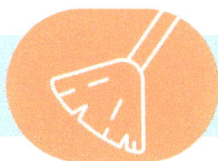

Laundry

The laundry room can be humid space where mold and mildew thrive. Using an essential oil formula to clean floors and walls could help eliminate this problem at the source. You could also add a few drops of essential oil to a humidifier to tackle musty odors. For pest infestation, use a strong essential oil spray to treat problem areas for spiders and other unwelcome visitors.

You will want to enhance your cleaning experience by adding essential oils to your laundry. Not only do they add a lovely fragrance to your wash, but essential oils help kill living organisms such as dust mites. We all hate to realize that dust mites live in our bedding, but they do – feeding on the dead skin cells we constantly shed. Recent studies have shown that eucalyptus oil kills dust mites. To effectively treat dust mites, experts suggest adding 25 drops of eucalyptus to each washing machine load, or approximately ½ ounce to a bottle of liquid detergent. Other essential oils you may want to add to the rinse cycle include fir, spruce, juniper, lavender, cedarwood, birch, or rosewood.

For the dryer, make your own dryer sheets by placing a

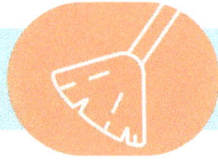

dampened washcloth with 10-12 drops of lavender, lemon, tea tree, bergamot, or another favorite essential oil in with the load. If hanging your laundry outside to air dry, spritz with a favorite essential oil!

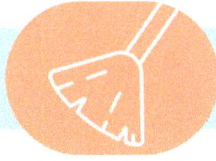

Stain Remover Spray for Clothes

What You Will Need:

2 tablespoons vegetable glycerin
2 tablespoons castile soap
¾ cup distilled water
10 drops lemon essential oil
8-ounce glass spray bottle

What To Do:

1. In a glass spray bottle, add all of the ingredients. Shake well.

2. To use, spray on stains before throwing in the wash. Be sure to check fabric for colorfastness before use.

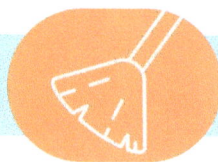

Basic Liquid Laundry Soap

Your laundry detergent can be customized with different essential oils based on your preference.

What You Will Need:

2 ¼ cups liquid castile soap
¼ cup white vinegar
¾ cup water
1 tablespoon glycerin
12 drops essential oil

What To Do:

1. In a large container, combine all of the ingredients and shake to blend.
2. Shake before use. To use, add a ¼ cup of liquid detergent per normal load. Use ½ cup for large or heavy loads.

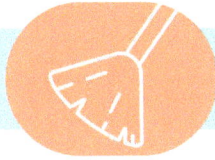

Rust Be Gone Stain Remover

Why pay too much for cleaners that don't work? Get rid of those hideous stains with this easy remedy.

What You Will Need:
5 drops lemon essential oil
½ cup lemon juice
¼ cup baking soda

What To Do:
1. Sprinkle the stain with baking soda, then add drops of essential oil and lemon juice.
2. Let sit overnight or several hours. Wipe baking soda solution away and rinse well.

- *Recipe variation:* Substitute another favorite essential oil such as orange in place of lemon essential oil.

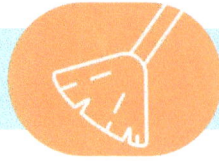

Stain-Off Spray

What You Will Need:
2 tablespoons borax
¼ cup oil-based soap
¼ cup glycerin
10 drops tea tree essential oil (or substitute: peppermint)
1 ¾ cups water
spray bottle

What To Do:

1. In a spray bottle, combine all of the ingredients. Shake well.
2. To use, spray generously on the stain. Wash as usual.

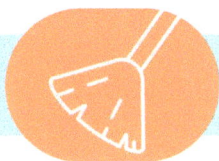

Basic Laundry Soap Powder

This recipe can be customized with your favorite essential oil.

What You Will Need:
2 cups baking soda
2 cups washing soda
1 cup soap flakes (or substitute: grated bar soap)
25 drops essential oil (your choice)
plastic container

What To Do:

1. In a large container, combine all of the ingredients. Stir well.
2. To use, add a ½ cup to wash for a normal-size load.

- *Note:* For hard water, add ½ cup borax and two cups of vinegar in a separate container and add ½ cup to wash.

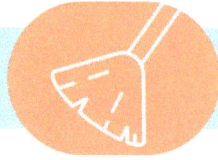

Spot-Off Stain Remover

When accidents happen, lift those stains off easily with this formula.

What You Will Need:

4 tablespoons cream of tartar
4 drops lemon essential oil (or substitute: peppermint)

What To Do:

1. In a small container, add all of the ingredients, along with a little water to create a paste.
2. To use, spread the paste over the affected area and allow to dry before throwing in the wash.

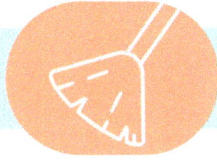

Fragrant Gel Air Freshener

Scented gel air fresheners are great for the laundry room, basement, or other rooms in the home.

What You Will Need:

1 tablespoon salt or 10-15 drops grain alcohol
2 tablespoons unflavored gelatin (2 packages)
1 cup water
10-15 drops essential oil
food coloring
salve containers or tins
small saucepan

What To Do:

1. Boil ½ cup of water, then add two envelopes of un-flavored gelatin. Stir to dissolve.
2. Add ½ cup of ice-cold water to gelatin mixture.
3. Add 10-15 drops of essential oil (any fragrance or blend you like).
4. Add 3-5 drops of food coloring.
5. Stir in a tablespoon of salt or 10-15 drops of alcohol, if used.
6. Pour gel mixture into 2-ounce tin containers. Allow to cool overnight (do not refrigerate).
7. To use, place open tins in a room, windowsill, in the car, etc.

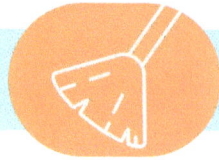

Dryer Sheets

These homemade dryer sheets are great for adding a fresh scent to your clothes.

What You Will Need:

1 cup vinegar
25 drops essential oil (i.e., orange, lemon, lavender)
cotton fabric (cut into squares)
2 mason jars

What To Do:

1. In a mason jar, combine vinegar and essential oils. Secure lid and shake to blend.

2. Place a cotton cloth into the vinegar mixture to absorb the liquid. Ring out excess liquid and place into another clean, dry jar with lid for storage. Repeat this process for each dryer sheet until all squares are saturated and then placed into the clean jar. If you have any leftover liquid, store in the mason jar with lid for a future batch.

3. To use, remove one dryer sheet and throw into dryer with load of clothes. The vinegar smell with evaporate in the dryer from the heat, leaving only the fresh scent of the oil.

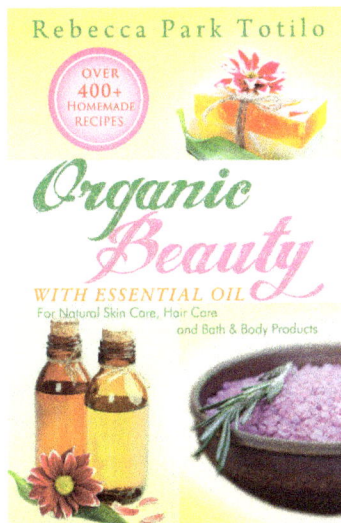

Organic Beauty With Essential Oil: Over 400+ Homemade Recipes for Natural Skin Care, Hair Care and Bath & Body Products

Sweep aside all those harmful chemically-based cosmetics and make your own organic bath and body products at home with the magic of potent essential oils! In this book, you'll find a luxurious array of over 400 Eco-friendly recipes that call for breathtaking fragrances and soothing, rich organic ingredients satisfying you head to toe. Included you'll find helpful can have the confidence knowing which essential oil to use and how much when creating your own body scrub, lip butter, or lotion bar! Discover how easy it is to make bath treats like fragrant shower gels, dreamy bubble baths, luscious creams and lotions, deep cleansing masks and facials for literally pennies using essential oils and ingredients from your kitchen.

145

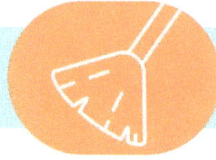

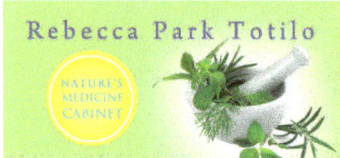

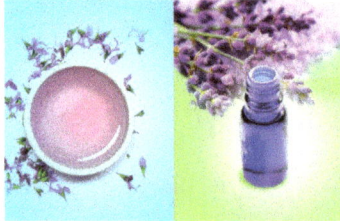

Heal With Essential Oil: Nature's Medicine Cabinet

Using essential oils drawn from nature's own medicine cabinet of flowers, trees, seeds and roots, man can tap into God's healing power to heal oneself from almost any pain. Find relief from many conditions and rejuvenate the body. With over 125 recipes, this practical guide will walk you through in the most easy-to-understand form how to treat common ailments with your essential oils for everyday living. Filled with practical advice on therapeutic blending of oils and safety, a directory of the most effective oils for common ailments and easy to follow remedies chart, and prescriptive blends for aches, pains and sicknesses.

Rebecca Park Totilo

OVER
170+
COMMON
AILMENTS

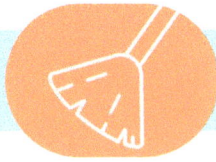

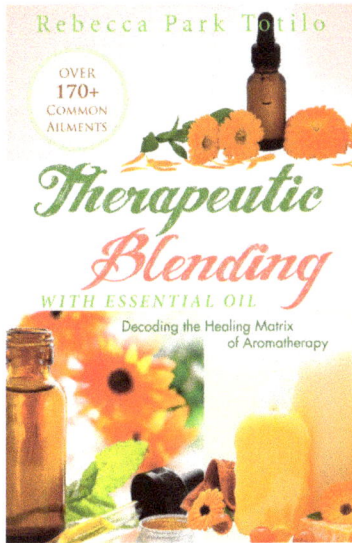

Therapeutic
Blending
WITH ESSENTIAL OIL
Decoding the Healing Matrix
of Aromatherapy

Therapeutic Blending With Essential Oil: Decoding the Healing Matrix of Aromatherapy

Therapeutic Blending With Essential Oil unlocks the healing power of essential oils and guides you through the intricate matrix of aromatherapy, with a compilation of over 170 common ailments. Discover how to properly formulate a blend for any physical or emotional symptom with easy to follow customizable recipes. Now, you can make your own massage oils, hand and body lotions, bath gels, compresses, salve ointments, smelling salts, nasal inhalers and more. This exhaustive guide takes all the guesswork out of blending oils from how many drops to include in a blend, to measuring thick oils, to how often to apply it for acute or chronic conditions. It also shows you how to create a single blend for multiple conditions. Even if you run out of oil for a favorite recipe, this book shows you how to substitute it with another oil.

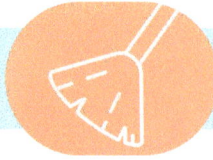

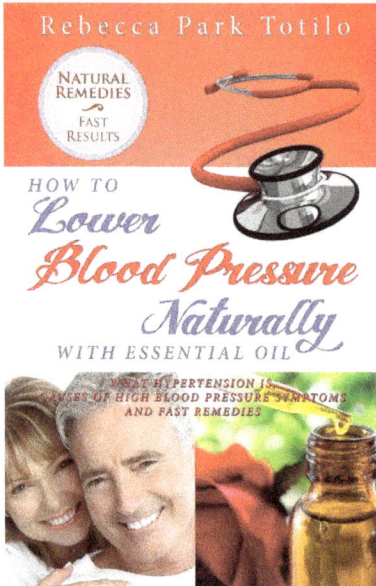

How To Lower Blood Pressure Naturally With Essential Oil: What Hypertension Is, Causes of High Pressure Symptoms and Fast Remedies

One out of three adults have it, and another one-third don't realize it. Oftentimes, it goes undetected for years. Even those who take multiple medications for it still don't have it under control. It's no secret -- high blood pressure is rampant in America. High blood pressure, or hypertension, has become a household term. Between balancing meds and monitoring diets though, are the true causes -- and best treatments -- hidden in the shadows? In How to Lower Blood Pressure Naturally With Essential Oil, Rebecca Park Totilo sheds light on what high blood pressure is, the causes and symptoms of high blood pressure, and which essential oils regulate blood pressure and how to use essential oils as a natural, alternative method.

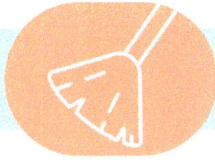

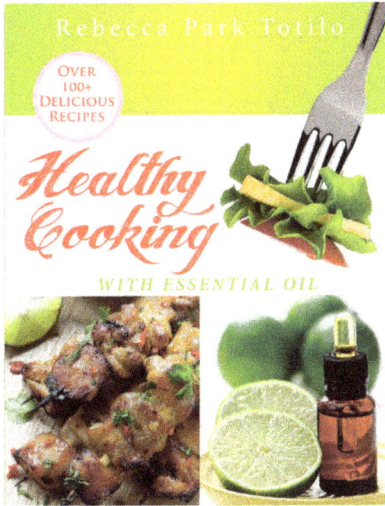

Healthy Cooking with Essential Oil

Imagine transforming an everyday dish into something extraordinary using only a drop or two of essential oil can enliven everything from soups, salads, to main dishes and desserts. Boasting flavor and fragrance, these intense essences can turn a dull, boring meal into something appetizing and delicious. Essential oils are fun, easy-to use and beneficial, compared to the traditional stale, dried herbs and spices found in most pantries today. Healthy food should never be thought of as mere fuel for the body, it should be enjoyed as a multi-sensory experience that brings therapeutic value as well as nourishment. For years we have limited the use of essential oils to scented candles and soaps, in the belief that they were unsafe to consume (and some are!). However, more people are realizing the value of using pure essential oils to enhance their diet. In Healthy Cooking With Essential Oil, you will learn how cooking with essential oils can open up a wealth of creative opportunities in the kitchen.

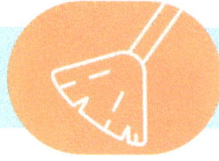

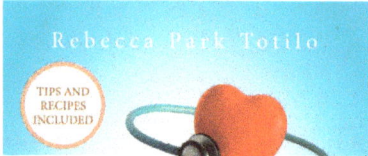

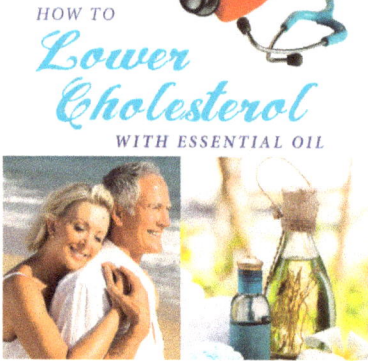

How to Lower Cholesterol with Essential Oil

Take healthy steps now to control high cholesterol and its risk factors with essential oils. People with high cholesterol have twice the risk for heart disease according to the Center for Disease Control and Prevention. What's worse, most folks aren't even aware that they have atherosclerosis until they have a heart attack or stroke. Lowering your cholesterol and triglycerides with essential oils may slow, reduce, or even stop the buildup of dangerous plaque in your arteries causing blockage of blood flow which could result in a heart attack or stroke. In this indispensable guide, author Rebecca Park Totilo presents scientific research supporting the efficacy of certain essential oils for lowering cholesterol, an extensive essential oil and carrier oil directory, natural treatments with recipes, along with easy-to-follow methods of use via inhalation, topically, and ingestion.

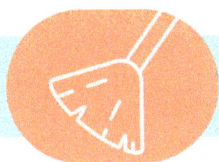

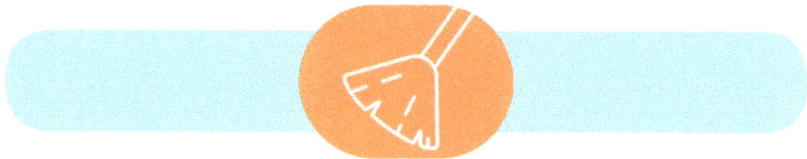